# Skin and Coat Care

BY LISA S. NEWMAN, N.D., Ph.D

Foreword by Deborah C. Mallu, D.V.M., C.V.A.

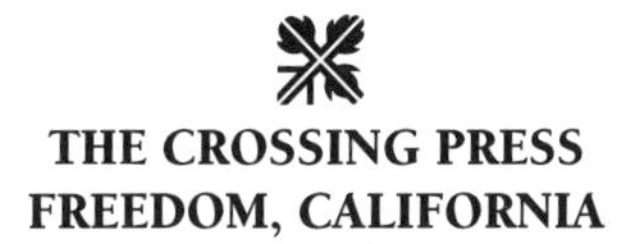

THE CROSSING PRESS
FREEDOM, CALIFORNIA

Cover photographs by Quarto, Inc. for Artville
Printed in the U.S.A.



For information on bulk purchases or group discounts for this and other Crossing Press titles, please contact our Special Sales Manager at 800/777-1048. Visit our web site: **www.crossingpress.com**

**Cautionary Note:** The nutritional information, recipes, and instructions contained within this book are in no way intended as a substitute for medical counseling. Please do not attempt self-treatment of a medical problem without consulting a qualified health practitioner.

The author and The Crossing Press expressly disclaim any and all liability for any claims, damages, losses, judgments, expenses, costs, and liabilities of any kind or injuries resulting from any products offered in this book by participating companies and their employees or agents. Nor does the inclusion of any resource group or company listed within this book constitute an endorsement or guarantee of quality by the author or The Crossing Press.

**Library of Congress Cataloging-in-Publication Data**

Newman, Lisa S.
Skin and coat care / by Lisa S. Newman.
p. cm. -- (The Crossing Press pocket series)
At head of title: Natural pet care.
ISBN 1-58091-008-4 (pbk.)
1. Dogs--Diseases--Alternative treatment. 2. Cats--Diseases--Alternative treatment. 3. Veterinary dermatology. 4. Holistic veterinary medicine. I. Title. II. Title: Natural pet care. III. Series.
SF992.S55N48 1999
636.7'08965--dc21 99-37375
CIP

# Contents

# Foreword

It is with great pleasure that I introduce Lisa Newman's remarkable series. She has dedicated her life to helping you care for your animal companions—we can all benefit from her years of experience.

We are living in a time of great change, especially in the realm of health care. As a practicing veterinarian for more than two decades, I have witnessed both myself and my clients begin to seek less invasive, more natural methods for healing our dogs and cats. Once we understood that all beings are interconnected on this planet, we became aware that our thoughts, emotions, and family dynamics played an important role in the health of our animal companions. We began to realize the importance of forming a team first with the members of our animal family, aided by other healing professionals including natural health counselors and animal communicators.

Over the years I have heard people say, "I didn't know you could use that natural remedy or treatment on animals." Feel confident that you can help your animal companions where the healing is best—in your loving home. Our animals nurture us by giving us unconditional love. In turn, we can nurture them with fresh, live food and supplements, so that they can live a long and healthy life. Lisa Newman will show you the way so that you can be empowered as a healer.

Deborah C. Mallu, D.V.M., C.V.A.

# What Does the Condition of Your Pet's Skin and Coat Tell You?

A luxurious coat and healthy firm skin are signs of your pet's vitality. Although topical treatments can make the skin and coat look healthy, there is no substitute for real fitness. Bright eyes, a good attitude, healthy digestion, and rapid recovery from a disease or an injury are signs of good health.

Many pet owners treat skin and coat conditions year after year with little long-term relief, and, as time passes, the symptoms usually become worse. Owners will try almost anything, including fancy hot oil treatments. They will eliminate substances that they believe are causing the problems. They will search for the another medication or change their pet's diet, but often, with each passing year the pet becomes weaker, the coat becomes less healthy, and skin inflammations are more frequent.

Allergies are often believed to cause most skin and coat conditions, but allergies are just another symptom and not the underlying problem. When the body is not cared for as nature intended, your pet's immune system grows weaker, which places extra stress on the body's other systems until the whole body breaks down. It is, therefore, not unusual to see the more serious diseases such as cancer in older animals with a history of skin and coat problems.

I believe that many symptoms are simply indications of imbalances in the immune system. Less than twenty percent of pets with suspected allergies have been correctly diagnosed. The remaining eighty percent have depressed immune systems and eat unbalanced diets.

Allopathic veterinarians, in general, tend to lump symptoms together under a general diagnosis and attempt to suppress symptoms, rather than treat the whole body.

Your pet's body is repeatedly bombarded by dangerous substances in the environment (for example, pesticides in the house), or in commercial pet food that contains animal by-products, rancid animal fat, and grain by-products (all common pet food ingredients). Waste builds up in the body, and the whole digestive system suffers. The skin, the body's largest eliminatory organ, then tries to release these wastes, which can result in pimples, rashes, and hot spots. Urea, a waste product of protein digestion, promotes a gout-like condition, which can cause a dull coat, foot chewing, and licking.

Steroids, commonly used to reduce inflammation, will temporarily reduce the symptoms by reducing the reaction to a toxin, but will not tackle the underlying problem of a depressed immune system. Though the symptoms appear to be reduced, the pet will not get better in the long run, and most animals will probably get worse.

To strengthen the immune system, it is necessary to cleanse the body of toxins. Supplements and homeopathic or herbal remedies will help to ensure that the fundamental imbalance is corrected. Feeding your pet at least twice a day and sometimes more if needed will help keep your pet's blood sugar stable and the hormonal system in balance. It is also important to provide proper grooming and an emotionally stable environment. You will find that this regime will foster a strong immune system and the symptoms will disappear.

The best defense for a pet with chronic symptoms is a strong offense. The first step is to get a proper diagnosis from your veterinarian to ensure that you are not dealing with a serious condition or disease. Holistic animal care is not to be used in lieu of, but as a support to veterinary care. Whatever the problem is, serious or minor, there are many natural protocols you can successfully follow.

Above all, do not give up prematurely. There are no magic bullets. Remember that the more compromised your pet's health is, and the longer he or she has suffered, the longer it will take to rebalance the body, but it is possible.

# Skin and Coat Conditions as Symptoms

Inbreeding, and excessive genetic manipulation of the more popular breeds, has minimized our animals' natural curative abilities, leaving them very susceptible to toxins. Years of vaccinations, chemical baths, flea and tick potions, dips and sprays, medications, and most importantly, poor-quality ingredients, artificial colors, preservatives, and by-products found in most pet foods and treats, all take their toll.

It is important to distinguish an isolated symptom from a depressed immune system. Although the holistic method of treatment is very similar in both cases, by defining toxins and understanding the relationship between waste products and the body's reaction to them, you will be better prepared to address your animal's individual needs and effectively reverse their condition, regardless of the cause.

The diagnosis of allergies has become too inclusive. Many poor skin and coat conditions, including digestive upsets, respiratory problems, arthritis, and poor immune function are often explained as allergic reactions. Some hypersensitivity reactions are true pathological processes that are triggered by the interaction of specific allergens, and the resulting symptom is caused by a true allergy.

Holistically, I see all skin and coat issues strictly as symptoms, rather than conditions. Even true allergies, whether the allergen is ingested, inhaled, or a chemical irritation, are typically just a form of hypersensitivity reaction. A specific allergic reaction is a symptom: Its underlying cause is rarely from the allergens themselves. Due to this difficulty of distinguishing between symptoms and causes, making a causative diagnosis and implementing a successful treatment protocol in chronic skin and coat conditions can be difficult.

Therapies that focus only on the removal of the allergen or the suppression of the body's reaction, rather than addressing the root cause, will give symptomatic relief at best. At worst, they will cause chronic, more frequent cycling of the symptoms, which places enormous burdens on the vital organs. This will happen even if the therapy you choose is a holistic one.

You must look beyond the symptoms or sensitivities. Certainly, I do not advocate allowing an animal to suffer from an oozing hot spot without addressing it. But, looking deeper, for the *cause* of the irritation, and *addressing that imbalance* will be more effective. It will dry up the hot spot faster, and may prevent it from re-occurring.

There are three most commonly diagnosed symptom types. You may be able to match your pet to one of these types; or you may have already received a similar diagnosis, possibly even one of "allergies." If you explore more deeply, you may find that the underlying cause is not a simple allergen. This deeper exploration may help you address your pet's symptoms more successfully, relieving them or reversing the sensitivity completely.

## DEFINING SYMPTOM TYPES

There are three types of irritants. The first are those that are inhaled by pets. Pets who have only airborne-related allergies, or whose skin and coat conditions are largely seasonal, are often diagnosed with sensitivities to inhaled allergens. Symptoms associated with inhaled allergens can include:

- general redness and itching of the skin with rashes or pustules (especially around the face, belly, and feet)
- hair loss and poor coat condition (brittle with dandruff or greasy)
- fur picking and poor coat growth or sheen

- ear or eye infections
- upper respiratory problems including asthma, excessive salivation, or nasal discharge
- irritability and a nervous nature, including restlessness at night with endless licking, biting, picking, and scratching.

Inhaled irritants are most often referred to as *airborne-related* symptoms. Pollen, dander, or dust causes these. Sources can vary from flowering trees and grasses, to your pet's own coat, to household dust. These can be the most frustrating conditions to deal with, because all too often it is virtually impossible to completely eliminate the source. If an allopathic treatment is adopted, animals seem to develop a tolerance to prescribed or over-the-counter antihistamines fairly quickly. Allergy shots, the most popular treatment for airborne sensitivities, often become less effective each season, leaving both owner and pet frustrated.

A holistic approach may prove successful for animals in this category. Elimination of the source is almost impossible because it will be extremely difficult to trace, and the traditional allopathic approach often results in an overall decline of health. There is a solution: Addressing the underlying imbalance of the immune system holistically quickly reverses most symptoms, and often completely eliminates the sensitivity to these allergens.

While symptom suppression alone can be successfully accomplished through natural methods, a *complete* holistic protocol of detoxification and nutritional and herbal supplementation is best. This protocol will stimulate the immune system, and lead to a more rapid and possibly more thorough reversal of the skin and coat conditions or sensitivities.

The second type of irritant resulting in skin and coat conditions is one caused by ingestion of foods or chemicals. Pets who have these symptoms are not predominantly affected by environmental or chemical toxins, such as pollen or dips, or by changes in the season. Ingested toxins can include individual foods and treats, and also by-products and chemicals in foods, such as preservatives and artificial flavors. These pets most often suffer from:

- skin, coat problems (including odor, hot spots, redness, and itching)
- gastric upset including bloating (the number one food-related acute cause of death in dogs)
- general loss of vitality
- vomiting, hair balls
- ear and eye discharges and irritation, especially in cats and small dogs
- gas, diarrhea and/or constipation, irritable bowel syndrome
- joint inflammation, muscular and arthritic pain
- organ failure
- excessive emotional/behavioral traits such as shyness, nervousness, or fear-aggression.

Ingested toxins are often thought to be *food allergies*. This is, in my opinion, the most misdiagnosed cause for skin and coat conditions. Chemical-based "allergies" are a close second. There are over thirty different commercial and prescription "skin and coat conditioning" or "allergy relief" diets, yet our pets are still suffering from dull coats, hot spots, diarrhea, constipation, irritable bowel syndrome, gas, and vomiting. Despite this plethora of "skin and coat" and "allergy-relief" diets, the symptoms continue because the true problem is the poor quality of the ingredients in our pets' food and the body's inability to digest and assimilate them.

Beef was one of the first ingredients targeted by veterinarians as a prime allergen or trigger for skin problems. Many pets that previously tested positive for beef sensitivity are now eating high-quality beef regularly with no symptoms.

Addressing food-related allergies holistically results in complete reversal of the symptoms in the majority of pets.

The third symptom type is caused by chemical irritation. Chemically irritated pets have a reaction to certain substances in their environment, including carpeting, shampoos, cigarette smoke, household cleaning products, vaccinations, pesticides, and even their own drinking water, beds, or collars. The body itself can produce chemical irritants, as in the case of hormones. Or there may be insufficient chemical output from the endocrine system, as in the case of cortisol deficiency. Stress on other glands, such as the thyroid or pituitary, may also result from or contribute to skin and coat problems and the general imbalances associated with them. There is a wide range of symptoms related to chemical irritants:

- poor coat condition including dry or greasy fur, coat loss, fur picking
- skin problems including dandruff, hot spots, pimples, redness, and itching
- ear and eye discharges and irritation
- gastric upset including bloating, as chemicals interfere with digestion
- gas, diarrhea and/or constipation, irritable bowel syndrome
- vomiting, hair balls
- general loss of vitality
- joint inflammation, muscular and arthritic pain
- organ failure from chronic symptoms such as F.U.S. (Feline Urological Syndrome), cystitis, diabetes, and even poor elimination
- excessive emotional/behavioral traits such as complete isolation, nervousness, fearfulness, or aggression
- seizures
- cataracts
- diabetes

- cancer, especially fatty skin tumors, sarcomas, and leukemia
- loss of reproductive capabilities
- general immune dysfunction

Chemically based sensitivities, also known as *environmental allergies*, are surprisingly common. Pets respond to their environment similar to the way we do. They react to the chemicals that pollute their bodies. Hair loss and skin rashes are common for pets exposed to environmental allergens. In some instances, our pets are exposed to far more chemicals than we ever are. Cats and dogs typically eat up to one-third their body weights in chemical preservatives each year, and they are completely doused in chemical pesticides, which are absorbed through the skin. When was the last time you took a bath in a lethal pesticide or wore a pesticide-laced collar daily?

Many pets spend a lot of time in direct contact with carpeting, floors, and outdoor landscapes that have been heavily treated with cleaning solutions, herbicides, and pesticides. This repeated exposure makes them more likely to develop sensitivities to these chemicals. Pets may spend their day outside breathing car exhaust, and their night inside, exposed to second-hand smoke. Even drinking water may be a culprit if it contains heavy metals, chemicals, bacteria, and amoebas. If you are not willing to drink your own tap water, then please do not give it to your animals.

Many pets may also suffer from multiple sensitivities, which cross between these major categories. Multiple symptoms and the resulting decline of health can be overwhelming. Traditionally, the allopathic approach has been to treat the various symptoms with a variety of drugs that may successfully suppress the symptom and temporarily alleviate suffering. But once medication is stopped, symptoms commonly recur and often worsen with each recurrence, even though the original cause (such as a carpet) has been removed.

It is impossible to affect one aspect of the body without affecting the rest. Chronic drug use may result in organ failure. Death can result from an ongoing assault on the body and the immune system. Too often, a pet is euthanized to end her or his suffering after drugs can no longer suppress the symptoms.

I do not advocate allowing an animal to suffer unnecessarily. I recommend using a medication prescribed by your veterinarian in the event of a *life-threatening* imbalance, infection, or injury. However, I do strongly urge that you change your pet's diet and improve his or her digestion and environment to strengthen its body first. Drugs should be seen as a last resort, warranted only in an emergency, as in the case of anaphylactic shock, adrenal malfunction, or a life-threatening staphylococcal infection. Consult with a veterinarian you trust, and weigh the pros and cons of various treatments.

# Assessing Skin and Coat Conditions

To assess of the nature of your pet's skin and coat condition by identifying a toxic reaction and its severity, you must incorporate information that includes:

- how acute (immediate) or chronic (long-term) the onset of symptoms is
- the time (i.e., after meals or early morning) or season in which it is most aggravated
- determining exposure to triggers in the environment or diet
- clinical tests

Skin tests and blood tests are used to confirm that the agents involved in an allergic reaction resulting in skin and coat conditions are present through the assessment of eosinophils, specific antibody levels, WBC (white blood cell) counts, histamine or other similar substances released.

When the veterinarian finds skin testing is contraindicated because of extreme dermatitis, the RAST (RadioAllergoSorbent Test) is performed. In this test, allergens are mixed with a sample of the animal's blood and the specific antibodies (and therefore the extent of the allergy) are determined. Although the results of these medical tests cannot be disputed, the veterinarian's response to these results and the recommended course of treatment, allopathic or holistic, can differ greatly.

The allopathic veterinary practitioner will often focus on the diagnosis of "allergies" and will seek to suppress symptoms through drugs (antihistamines, antibiotics, steroids for inflammation and some immune stimulation). Based on test results, the veterinarian will attempt to identify the specific allergens responsible, so that they may be avoided. But all too often, shortly upon the termination of medication, there is a full return of symptoms.

The holistic practitioner, on the other hand, will use these tests as confirmation of an underlying imbalance. Initially, certain ingredients which have tested positive as an allergen may be avoided, and certain symptoms suppressed (preferably naturally). Emphasis is placed on stimulating the immune system into reversing the poor skin and coat condition, thereby eliminating the symptoms. In a large percentage of animals, holistic animal care allows the reintroduction of the very ingredients previously known to have triggered an allergic response.

## ALLERGIES, SENSITIVITIES, OR TOXICITY?

Let us now explore and evaluate what a true allergy is, and determine how often sensitivities or even toxicity are the true culprits behind that so-called "allergic" reaction. In my experience, there is an overemphasis by veterinarians and pet storeowners on allergy symptoms rather than on investigating *why* and *how* the body reacts as it does. Often, the animal's symptoms are cyclic, fluctuating from diet to diet, or from one conditioner to another, with medications (including allergy shots) used to suppress the resulting symptoms. With each cycle or season, the allergy response becomes worse and more difficult to treat. Tests are performed to identify specific allergens and every attempt is made to avoid these sources. Short-term relief is generally successful, as long as the body remains responsive to medication. Eventually, more serious allergies and other progressive diseases can develop.

Sophisticated skin and blood tests may be able to ascertain what is happening with the body's biochemical processes, but unfortunately, they rarely identify a true allergen. Only detective work on the part of the owner will uncover the culprit.

Blood work identifies the presence of various markers, such as histamine, lymphocytes, and antibodies to specific allergens (i.e., beef proteins). These markers indicate that the immune system has marshaled a defense. It does not show us if the specific source is the actual allergen, or whether a toxic level of waste *from that source* is the allergen. For example, if beef protein is compromised (i.e., diseased tissue or non-digestible sources such as hide or hooves) and the body has a difficult time digesting and assimilating it, then a higher quantity of waste product will circulate in the blood. These toxins could also trigger a release of histamines, but the blood work would only reveal that beef is the allergen. A standard course of treatment would recommend the elimination of beef and beef by-products. This same pet, supported holistically and presented with a higher-quality beef diet, will no longer exhibit symptoms.

This dilemma is at the crux of the allergy firestorm and other chronic symptom conditions. In holistic circles, this process is known as a "sensitivity." For example, if your body is constantly covered in filth, it will eventually begin to respond to the filth; possibly resulting in the skin tissues becoming sensitive and irritated. Imagine that the body is submersed in a vat of filth ten hours per day, and the prescribed treatment for the resultant skin problems was a fifteen-minute shower and the application of medicated creams two or three times per day. How quickly do you think the skin would heal completely? Would it ever have a chance to completely heal, being exposed daily, for hours at a time to the source of irritation?

The same holds true for filth inside the body. It remains in contact with the mucous membranes in the respiratory or the digestive tract, irritating the nervous system, weakening the immune system and causing imbalances in the glandular system. The eliminatory system becomes overburdened and unable to filter (detoxify) this filth.

As a holistic practitioner, I fully understand this vicious cycle and why it occurs in so many pets today. Our pets are constantly bombarded with chemicals, by-products, vaccinations, etc., and subjected to life in a symbolic "vat" of filth. When a substance is not easily decomposed, absorbed, and eliminated by the body, waste accumulates. An overabundance of waste results in toxic levels, which stimulates the immune system to release agents to corral and eliminate the culprit (hence, the positive results in blood work-ups). Waste is also eliminated through the skin, causing it to become symptomatic. But the condition cannot be reversed through repeated suppression of symptoms with chemical treatment. This cycle of symptom suppression and recurrence sentences thousands of pets to a lifetime of pain and suffering and perpetuates the myth that "allergies" cannot be cured.

## THE UNDERLYING IMBALANCE

The diagnosis of "allergies" has steadily increased over the past ten years. In 1986 a valuable book identified several important factors to aid in the understanding and treatment of allergy sensitivities. In *Pet Allergies: Remedies for an Epidemic*, Alfred J. Plechner, DVM, and Martin Zucker described how commercial pet food ingredients can undermine general health. The authors also emphasized the negative results of improper breeding practices, which create genetically crippled animals and rampant disease. They discussed the safe use of steroids and hormones in specific cases. For the most part, veterinarians and breeders for whom the book was written ignored it.

Pet food companies have manufactured new and improved diets for allergy symptoms based on new sources of animal protein instead of the traditional beef, meat meal and bone meal, pork by-products, and other animal by-products. Unfortunately, these new sources are not too different from the old: lamb, lamb meal and bone meal, poultry by-products, fish by-products and "other" animal by-products! The use of chemicals in pet foods is still rampant. If anything, there are even more chemicals and by-products being fed to our pets today under the guise of a "natural" or "anti-allergen" product! The fundamental quality of the diet is still sadly lacking.

Breeders continue to breed animals known to have a predisposition towards allergies. Veterinarians continue to use Prednisone, antihistamines, and antibiotics, but misunderstand the true benefit of these medications in some allergy-related cases. Plechner and Zucker describe how the use of corticosteroids can reestablish cortisol levels (a deficiency of which is seen in many allergy-suffering pets), which stimulates and strengthens the immune system, and promotes reversal of skin and coat symptoms. They suggested simple blood work that could be used to determine which animals could truly profit from steroids (to reverse a deficiency), and which animals would benefit from hormone therapy, instead of using the shotgun approach and giving these medications to any pet with similar symptoms. This method of identification is extremely helpful in those pets with true deficiencies that *should* be treated chemically. In those animals without true deficiencies, the immune system could be stimulated naturally through nutritional, herbal, and homeopathic supplementation, rather than further burdened by medications *not truly needed.*

The quality and freshness of the ingredients in food play a role in triggering many skin and coat conditions. It is not necessarily the ingredient itself that is the culprit. Certainly, one should always seek to eliminate a food ingredient which may be an allergen, but a greater focus on the body's ability to properly digest and assimilate nutrition, eliminate waste, and repair and maintain healthy cells for a strong immune system is essential to the elimination of your pet's poor skin and coat condition.

Even if medication is needed, your pet's lifestyle can be enriched through holistic animal care. You will succeed if you honor life as nature's gift to your animal and use a holistic style to fully realize your pet's self-curative potential.

# What is Holistic Animal Care?

Rather than simply addressing an animal's symptoms, holistic animal care addresses the whole body: body, mind, spirit, and even the environment. Different health modalities are used in a synergistic way to help stimulate, strengthen, and support the body's own biological processes and natural defenses.

Nutrition, which can often be the deciding factor between health and disease, is central to holistic care. It doesn't matter what number of drugs or natural remedies are given to a pet, if the pet is not receiving adequate nutrition, it will be lacking the basic tools with which to support its own recovery.

Nutrition is also the cornerstone of a modality known as naturopathy. Defined by a medical dictionary as "a drugless system of therapy by the use of physical forces, such as air, light, water, heat, massage, etc.," naturopathy is a comprehensive approach that emphasizes supporting the body's physical attempts to eliminate disease. Naturopaths believe that a major cause of disease is an excessive buildup of toxic materials (often due to improper eating and lack of exercise) which clog the eliminatory system. Various techniques are used to clean out (detoxify) the body and stimulate reversal of symptoms and disease. The cleansing process is supported with high-quality nutrition, proper food combining (to stimulate and aid digestion), nutritional supplements, and herbs.

Herbs have been widely used by every culture since ancient times to stimulate healing. It is widely believed that people began using herbs after observing wild animals that instinctively select appropriate herbs when they are ill. Herbalists use specific herbal leaves, roots, bark, flowers, and seeds to assist the healing process, primarily by helping detoxify the body. Herbs provide a slower and deeper action than do pharmaceutical drugs.

Another modality, which also provides a slower and deeper action, is homeopathy. Sometimes nutrition or herbs can begin the cleansing process and support the body so that it can cure itself. But often it is the homeopathic remedy, which can stimulate the deeper levels of healing. The homeopathic system is safe, its basic principles are elegantly simple, and homeopathic remedies have been exhaustively researched and used successfully for hundreds of years.

The German physician, Samuel Hahnemann, founded homeopathy in the late 1700s. It is based on the principle, "Like will cure like." The ancient Chinese masters of the healing arts, Hindu sages, as well as our history's most noted physicians and alchemists, Hippocrates and Paracelsus, recognized this principle. Hahnemann's "provings"—that a substance that can mimic symptoms helps cure as well—revolutionized the understanding of symptoms and disease. Trained as a physician, Hahnemann treated symptoms as unhealthy responses of the body that should be suppressed. He later learned that symptoms can be positive, adaptive responses to stresses that the body experiences. Hahnemann recognized that symptoms represented the body's effort to heal itself, and therefore our aim should be to stimulate, rather than suppress, the body's own defenses.

Hahnemann noted certain similarities between symptoms produced by some diseases and by the very drugs used to treat them. From this he formed his "Law of Similars," postulating that a disease could be cured by whatever medicine produces similar symptoms when given to a healthy person. The beauty of homeopathic treatment is that it cooperates, rather than competes, with the body's own efforts to regain health.

A simplified example of how homeopathy works is that of bee venom. We know that a bee sting will cause swelling, fluid accumulation, redness of the skin, pain, and soreness that is accentuated by the application of heat or pressure. Sensitive animals will also experience mental (emotional) symptoms such as apathy, stupor, listlessness, or the opposite, whining and fearfulness. If a homeopathically prepared dilute solution of bee venom (known as Apis) is given to a pet with these symptoms—even if the symptoms are caused by something other than a bee sting—the condition will soon begin to clear up. The key is that the symptoms are quite similar to what the remedy, in its undiluted state, would create. Flower essences (which balance emotional states) and tissue cell salts (which support physiological processes) act similarly, by stimulating the body's own natural healing and homeostasis.

## THE HOLISTIC PET

A healthy, holistically reared pet is in a state of balance that exists on three interrelated levels: the physical, the emotional, and the environmental. A healthy pet experiences physical vitality and is free from physiological malfunction, displays emotional clarity resulting in good behavior and happiness, and receives (as well as contributes) joy, love, and security in their living environment.

This animal is the opposite of a chemically reared pet, who is often found to be in a state of imbalance or dis-ease. This animal lacks physical vitality and suffers from chronic symptoms due to physiological malfunction, displays emotional stress resulting in negative behavior, and often also lives in a physically toxic environment. Since it is impossible to have one organ system affected without it affecting the other organ systems, a system that is not in balance is more susceptible to assault.

Holistic animal care is simple and safe to use. *Treat the body well and the body will be well.* By providing the body with sufficient amounts of high-quality food, correct supplements, and holistic modalities when appropriate, the body will remain in a state of balance. If certain substances, which create an imbalance, assault the balanced body, it has the strength to trigger the curative process and reestablish its homeostasis.

## SKIN AND COAT PROBLEMS

Some pets who develop allergies to particular foods are born genetically compromised. Other pets, who were not born genetically compromised, suffer from skin and coat problems due to exposure to chemicals, or an emotionally and/or physically toxic environment. Chemicals alter the body's primary biological functions, place undue stress on vital organs and glands necessary for proper immune function, and destroy healthy tissue. Pets with skin and coat problems have often been exposed to:

- standard commercial pet foods
- artificial treats
- shotgun medications (the indiscriminate use of "standard" medications)
- excessive vaccinations and yearly boosters
- toxic cleaning and pest control products (especially collars or monthly drug doses)
- environmental pollution (without the benefit of regular detoxification)
- an emotionally and/or physically stressful living environment (past and present)

## COMMERCIAL FOODS INCREASE SUSCEPTIBILITY TO SKIN AND COAT SYMPTOMS

Commercial pet diets and treats are the primary reason pets develop all types of inflammatory responses, including food allergies, which can cause skin and coat problems. It should be noted that the quality of the ingredients can do more harm and is more likely to trigger a response than the ingredients themselves. The standard use of by-products and meat sources unfit for human consumption severely limits the pet's ability to digest and assimilate nutrients well. The use of artificial colors or flavors, chemical preservatives, nitrates, and rancid animal fats also interferes with digestion. Poorly digested matter becomes harder to eliminate, causing a backup of old fecal material in the bowel, which further prohibits assimilation of vital nutrients.

Pets often don't get enough exercise and aren't given the opportunity to go outside to move their bowels. An animal who is fed a poor diet filled with chemicals and by-products will not be able to properly digest the food. This undigested matter moves into the colon, but since complete evacuation is not really possible, old fecal material will line the walls of the colon. Chemicals (such as ethoxyquin, a commonly used pet food preservative that is a moisture prohibitive) limit the lubrication necessary for a properly evacuated stool, and the fecal material hardens, finally producing small, hard, dry stools.

Most companies state that their pet food is "more digestible with less waste," but what do you think a physician would say to you if you described your own stools as small, hard lumps? Certainly, a better-quality food will produce less stool volume (generally due to less fillers, and better digestibility), but it should not be caused by the lack of moisture in the stool. The colon requires ample hydration to function properly, so it is very important to provide fresh, filtered drinking water.

As old fecal material builds up inside the colon, it becomes harder and harder for the body to clean out this material on its own. This interferes with the body's ability to absorb nutrients from digested matter in the colon into the bloodstream for distribution to the body's hungry cells and energy-depleted organ systems.

The harder the ingredients are to break down and process, and the more chemicals present, the more stress is placed on the body. The harder the body has to work, the quicker it breaks down. Due to improper digestion and assimilation, the body lacks the resources to utilize whatever nutrients are provided. Improper digestion and assimilation also leads to a build-up of general waste (toxins) in the body, placing a huge burden on the eliminatory organs. As the liver and kidneys become overburdened, the body attempts to detoxify through the largest eliminatory organ, the skin. Hence, skin and coat problems emerge. Additionally, the lymph system and endocrine system are over-stimulated, possibly leading to the development of a deeper, more serious disease, such as cancer.

## CHEMICALS IN SUBSTANCES OTHER THAN FOOD INGREDIENTS

A pet may also be exposed to chemicals and irritants in other, non-dietary forms. Whether the irritant is a chemical-based breath mint given as a treat, an annual vaccination booster, an artificially perfumed shampoo, a medicated skin treatment, flea or tick control products, household cleaning agents, or long-term medication, any or all can have a detrimental effect on your animal's health. If you think of the healthy body as a balanced scale, when you continually add chemicals to one side of the scale, it will remain out of balance, but if you add good nutrition and minimize the build-up of chemicals, the scale remains in balance.

## OTHER FACTORS CREATING IMBALANCE IN A PET

It is important to recognize and address other factors that

may cause imbalance and interfere with homeostasis. Structural imbalances are often a prime cause of dis-ease. Old injuries or genetic malfunctions, such as rheumatoid arthritis, can place stress on certain organ systems. A build-up of calcium deposits and joint or spinal inflammation may also put pressure on nerves involved with digestive organs, such as the stomach. This pressure can interfere with the normal function of the stomach and lead to improper digestion and assimilation of nutrients. Often, addressing the structural problems will help to reverse the poor skin and coat condition. Chiropractic adjustments, massage, acupressure, and acupuncture can all be beneficial tools to alleviate your animal's symptoms.

Another issue that can cause imbalance is a stressful environment. Have you ever "felt butterflies in your stomach" and experienced a loose bowel movement due to a stressful situation? Pets who often experienced extreme emotions (fear, nervousness, and tension) are also more likely to suffer from digestive problems and glandular imbalances, which may exacerbate skin and coat symptoms, especially shedding and obsessive fur pulling. Sources of environmental stress include family changes such as relocating, members leaving or dying, divorce, new births, or new jobs, etc. The pituitary, adrenal, and thyroid glands may be injured by chronic emotional stress. These glands are associated with the "fight or flight" reaction to negative stimuli. A safe and nurturing environment will ensure your pet's emotional well-being. The use of nutritional supplementation and remedies, especially flower essences, to rebalance the emotions can often be the key to a more complete physical healing.

When an animal is out of balance, waste builds up not only in the colon but also in the bloodstream and eliminatory organs. Urea, a waste product of meat protein metabolism, can cause skin-related conditions and also accounts for the large number of pets who test positive for meat allergies. The poorer the quality of meat and the more difficult it is to digest, the more waste is produced during digestion. Urea toxicity manifests itself in certain, notable symptoms:

- known or suspected allergies to beef, pork, meat, meat by-products, or meat meal
- excessive licking and chewing of paws, resulting in lick granuloma
- prickly heat-type rashes, itchy skin, with or without small pimples or pustules
- excessive loss of hair or coat condition
- foul-smelling breath, flatulence, and/or stool
- increased fatty tumor, cyst, or cancerous tumor production
- liver, pancreas, gall bladder, and kidney dysfunction
- weakened immune responses, especially chronic skin infections
- premature aging with or without chronic muscular pain and/or arthritic symptoms
- parasitic infestation, especially fleas and ticks (which feed off skin-eliminated waste)
- neurological problems, including seizures
- aggression and other behavioral problems

Yeast, another nasty ingredient, is found in the majority of commercial pet diets, treats, supplements, flea and tick control products, and even many pet medications. Yeast, which is noted for its anti-flea and tick properties, is in practically everything! A cheap filler ingredient, it does provide some B vitamins, minerals, amino acids, and natural flavor to products, but is mostly used to increase the food's volume.

The most common form of yeast found in animal products is brewer's yeast, which is a waste product that has most of its nutrients eliminated during the brewing process. Yeast was long touted as a good source of nutrients, but we are now finding that this is not so. Nutritional yeast, a cultivated product, is nutritionally superior to brewer's yeast and tastier, but it still is not the best source of nutrients and, like brewer's yeast, it can be difficult to digest. Adequate levels of B vitamins are only available through supplements. It would take far too much yeast to provide an equivalent amount. Moreover, excessive yeast clogs the liver and increases general toxicity. According to recent veterinary research, animals are more likely to be allergic to yeast than to most other food sources.

Humans, too, do not digest yeast well. Poor digestion places an additional burden on the liver, resulting in skin conditions. Chinese medicine recognizes the correlation between the liver and the skin. Yeast supplementation, which is prescribed by vets and alternative practitioners, is the culprit. Yeast may initially improve pets' skin, but the pets' symptoms often become more intense and more difficult to treat, which can cause liver toxicity symptoms. I always recommend detoxification and the total elimination of yeast and sugar (which compounds yeast toxicity) from animals' diets for six weeks. Other than a daily multiple vitamin/mineral supplement (high in B vitamins) nothing else is used to treat pets' skin conditions, yet it will quickly resolve on its own.

Yeast toxicity manifests itself in certain symptoms, most notably:

- slower healing of skin problems
- excessive loss of fur or coat condition
- excessive licking and chewing of the body and face rubbing
- hot spots, itchy skin, with or without small pimples or pustules
- foul-smelling breath, flatulence and/or stool (especially off-colored stool with mucus)
- known or suspected allergies to yeast or yeast-containing foods such as dry kibble

- ear infections, eye discharges, and upper respiratory problems, including asthma
- increased fatty tumor, cyst, or cancerous tumor production
- poor digestion and assimilation of other nutrients
- blood sugar instability
- high levels of liver enzymes and eosinophils (represents a damaged liver)
- liver, spleen, gall bladder, and/or pancreatic dysfunction including diabetes
- weakened immune responses, especially chronic skin infections
- premature aging with or without digestive symptoms
- increased sensitivities to pollution, vaccinations, and chemicals in general
- aggression, fearful-aggressive, or fearful behavior in certain pets
- parasitic infestation, especially fleas and ticks (who feed off of skin-eliminated waste)

As urea, metabolized yeast, and other excess waste builds up in the body, undue stress is placed upon vital organs. First, the ability to break down nutrients is reduced, waste begins to circulate, and fewer nutrients are available to stimulate the body's defenses. Next the eliminatory, lymphatic, and immune systems become burdened. Chronic symptoms develop—notably those diagnosed as "allergies"—and suppression of the symptoms is initiated. Once medication is stopped, the symptoms return and the cycle continues. Ultimately, there is organ and gland malfunction, possibly leading to an early death.

Any pet suffering from parasitic infestations, sensitivities, or toxicity can benefit from holistic animal care. Regardless of the symptoms, the underlying causes are fundamentally the same. A wholesome, toxin-free approach to diet and environment can not only prevent an apparent symptom, but can also reverse it more quickly and effectively than the further application of chemicals.

# Holistic Care of Skin and Coat Conditions

To reverse the symptoms that can manifest as skin and coat conditions, a holistic animal care lifestyle should be followed or there is the risk that symptoms will only be suppressed temporarily. Fasting and detoxification is an important first step. These processes help prepare the body for further re-balancing, and ultimately for healing. Changing to a natural, high-quality diet, supplemented with nutritional, herbal, and homeopathic products, provides the necessary foundation to stimulate your pet's natural healing ability.

Treating skin and coat conditions without first addressing a possible underlying nutritional imbalance is a waste of time. Diet may be a causative factor. Many treats, and even so-called "natural" supplements, are full of fillers such as yeast, chemicals, artificial flavors, and colors. Look carefully at what you are feeding your pet. Re-balance a home-cooked diet, or find a better-quality commercial diet, and your pet's poor condition may be reversed.

To introduce a dietary change and initiate a successful program to relieve your pet's skin and coat conditions, begin by imposing a short twenty-four hour period of fasting. Many people associate fasting with deliberately starving their pet. Yet this couldn't be farther from the truth. Fasting can save your pet's life!

Fasting encourages the body to detoxify and re-balance. Old fecal material is expelled from the colon. Vital eliminatory organs—the kidneys and liver—are given a respite from processing waste, thus allowing a deeper processing of backed-up toxins to take place. Digestion and elimination, necessary processes for the uptake of nutrients and therapeutic substances such as herbs, are improved. The immune system, which helps the body resist toxins, is strengthened and the overall condition of your pet is improved.

The fasting methods we will explore are very safe and gentle. People are bothered most when their pets look at them pleadingly at dinnertime. It is true that twenty-five percent of that pleading look may be caused by hunger, but the other seventy-five percent is an attempt to control you. Pets, particularly dogs, are experts at controlling their masters. To avoid the pleading look during fasting, do something with your pet at their usual dinnertime that is fun. Bring home a new kitty toy (but, please not out of guilt!), or take your canine friend out for a fifteen-minute walk. These activities will not only occupy you and your pet's minds, but will also provide you both with exercise. If fasting is not appropriate for your pet because of her or his physical condition, homeopathic detoxification works well by itself.

In order to encourage more efficient elimination during the twenty-four hour period of fasting, you can add a homeopathic remedy. This combination of fasting along with a homeopathic remedy is the best detoxification method. If you use the homeopathic remedy or the fasting alone, the process will take longer.

Anyone who has tried to clean with a dirty sponge knows that a clean sponge does a more efficient job. Even a short twenty-four hour fast with homeopathic support can make a world of difference. Detoxification makes for better digestion and better assimilation of the vital nutrients necessary to help stimulate healing and strengthening. Without proper detoxification, the body's ability to cure itself is limited.

Once the overall detoxification process has occurred, usually within the first six to eight weeks, you will see a reversal of symptoms. In over seventy-five percent of cases I have observed, this method of detoxification, along with dietary changes and basic nutritional support, effectively ended the pet's suffering.

In the remaining twenty-five percent of cases, including those with true allergies or chronic debilitating dis-ease, the judicious use of homeopathic, herbal, and nutritional supplementation in a continuing course of treatment will definitely strengthen your animal's constitution and reduce, or eventually eliminate, their condition. With these cases, it can often take a few years for the body to eliminate the skin and coat conditions completely.

Treating your pet's toxic reactions holistically, rather than relying on symptom suppression, is the quickest, most effective way to reverse a symptom or any underlying condition completely. With a systematic detoxification and strengthening program, the underlying condition will progressively improve, but the improvement may be subtle. Don't stop detoxification and supplementation as soon as symptoms have been suppressed because the body can become burdened again, since it has a predisposition to this weakness, and will again respond to toxins, allergens, or stress.

For pets with true allergies or chronic dis-ease, the results of an ongoing holistic animal care program can be miraculous. As each year passes, the body will become stronger and less sensitive to allergens and toxins. With each year, your pet will exhibit less severe symptoms, they become easier to treat, and there will be faster resolution. In those animals that are genetically or environmentally predisposed to deeper dis-ease, holistic animal care will minimize the possibility of degenerative conditions and maximize healing potential.

Before starting a fasting program, check with your veterinarian. Perhaps your pet has diabetes and must maintain his or her blood sugar with food as well as insulin. Perhaps your veterinarian feels that your pet is too weak to fast, or your pet has had a recent bout of minor infections. It is always wise to rely on a trusted medical opinion, especially if you have a veterinarian who supports your holistic lifestyle.

There are two methods to fasting I recommend. The major factor to consider when deciding which fasting method is best for your pet is your pet's condition prior to starting the fast.

## THE STANDARD FAST

The standard method is used for pets with acute or chronic symptoms that are otherwise in good health, and can adhere to a straight fast. Age makes no difference, as I have seen fasting succeed with a struggling one-week-old kitten or a 14-year-old dog.

### Day One

Feed breakfast as you normally would on the morning you are to begin the fast. Eliminate the evening meal. Be sure to provide plenty of fresh, pure drinking water. Provide fun-filled activity in fresh air and sunshine, twice during the first day, followed by a damp terry cloth rubdown. Be sure not to overtire or place undue stress on your pet.

### Day Two—Breaking the Fast

The following morning (after twenty-four hours of fasting) feed your pet one-half its usual breakfast. To make this process really special, break the fast with cooked oatmeal. It will absorb impurities in the digestive tract. To the oatmeal, you can add a teaspoon or two of raw honey, encapsulated garlic oil (raw garlic can be too harsh at this point), and some type of fresh green extract such as barley grass or spirulina. A fresh green extract can be very soothing and cleansing to the digestive tract after fasting. Cats may prefer a little tuna water for flavor. Supplements can also be added back into the diet at this time.

Provide exercise in the fresh air and sunshine twice on this second day, followed by a damp terry cloth rubdown. Remember plenty of water and be sure not to overtire or stress out your pet. For dinner, feed the normal quantity (and, hopefully, better quality) of food.

This is also a good fasting protocol to follow on a weekly basis to help maintain general health and well-being, especially in dogs. Cats may prefer to regulate their own fasting periods. Regarding this weekly fast, you will quickly find what suits you and your own animal's needs. Remember that exercise is very important at all times, but is especially important during cleansing to help move toxins out of the body by stimulating the eliminatory organs. The terry cloth rubdown helps to stimulate the skin as it continues to process waste from the body's detoxification. If an odor is present during fasting, mix one-quarter cup of baking soda to one gallon of warm, purified water, rinse your pet's body with this solution, and dry it with a towel. The baking soda will help to neutralize the odor and balance the skin's pH, reducing any itching. Avoid using tap water, as it contains chlorine (a known skin irritant that will increase itching), which will be reabsorbed into the skin. If tap water is the only available water, boil it for fifteen minutes to help evaporate the chlorine. Be sure to let it cool down before using. A cut-up lemon boiled in the water for twenty minutes, then strained, acts as an additional deodorizer and disinfectant.

Generally, a standard twenty-four hour fast is sufficient, but you may choose to follow it for two to three days longer if your pet was suddenly overcome by allergies, is fighting an infection, has been on very poor-quality diets, or has not been eating well.

## EXTENDED STANDARD FAST

### Day One

Use the same protocol as the standard fast.

### Day Two (and possibly Day Three, Day Four)

Provide fun-filled activity in fresh air and sunshine twice during this day of fasting, followed by a damp terry cloth rubdown. Be especially careful not to overtire or place undo stress on your pet. Apple juice or vegetable juices (carrot, celery, or parsnip is best—avoid tomato juice) may be given in small amounts during the day, approximately one-quarter cup per twenty-five pounds of body weight per day. Do not over-do! These juices can also be frozen into small ice cubes for your pet's enjoyment during warmer months.

### Breaking Fast Day

Break the fast with one-quarter of your pet's normal quantity of food in the morning, and the same (one-quarter) quantity for dinner. Both meals should be the cooked oatmeal. A little fruit or vegetable fiber (from juicing) also can be added to the oatmeal and future meals.

### Second Day of Breaking Fast

Feed one-half normal rations in the morning and evening of the second day. Mix your pet's new natural diet fifty-fifty with cooked oatmeal.

### Third Day of Breaking Fast

Feed full rations of a natural diet of your choice at breakfast and dinner. This is a good time to introduce fresh fruits and vegetables to your pet's diet on a regular basis.

## THE ALTERNATIVE FASTING METHOD

An alternative fasting method may be more appropriate for pets with general symptoms that also struggle with other serious conditions, such as cancer or diabetes, or are initially very debilitated and require additional nutritional and/or herbal support. To avoid huge dips in blood sugar and additional stress on the animal's biochemical balance, fasting should be limited to twenty-four hours. Actually, it is easier and almost as beneficial for the body to complete several twenty-four hour fasts within a few weeks, even if there are only a few days break between each twenty-four hour fast, rather than fasting for three or four consecutive days.

### Day One

Feed your pet her or his usual breakfast. For the evening meal substitute a vegetable broth. To make this broth, grate equal amounts of fresh, raw carrots, beets, parsley, parsnips, spinach, and kale to make up a total of one cup of combined vegetables. Add grated vegetables to four cups of boiling water (avoid tap water) and simmer on low until all the vegetables are very soft, about twenty to thirty minutes. Separate the cooked vegetables and refrigerate to be used later. Refrigerate the broth in a well-sealed container.

Feed your pet one-half cup of broth per twenty pounds of body weight, per meal. You may give one or two additional meals of this broth during the fasting, if your animal seems to be very hungry, but do not overfeed in one sitting. Prior to feeding, warm the broth—but never in the microwave which will destroy any available nutrients. Cold broth may upset sensitive stomachs and lacks palatability. Prior to feeding the broth, give your pet orally any supplements or medications prescribed to be given with food.

### Break Alternative Fast Day

The next morning feed your pet one-half the amount of broth you used during the preceding day, adding one-quarter the normal ration of food. Cooked oatmeal may be a good alternative to regular food during this fast-breaking period, especially if there is a lot of colon cleansing needed. Repeat morning menu for the evening meal.

### Second Day of Breaking the Alternative Fast

Feed one-half the amount of broth you used during the fast and add one-quarter the normal ration of food or one-eighth ration of food and one-eighth ration of cooked oatmeal. For the evening meal feed three-quarters the normal ration of food (no broth).

### Third Day of Breaking the Alternate Fast

Introduce the full ration of your pet's natural diet at each meal.

This protocol will allow the body to begin detoxification without excess stress. When in doubt as to which process you should follow, it might be best to use the alternative fasting protocol. In a pinch, try cutting back twenty-five to fifty percent of your pet's standard meal with the addition of nutritional supplements, herbal extracts, vegetable and fruit juices—which will also serve to stimulate a deeper elimination, without upsetting your pet's metabolism.

## HERBS

Listed below are the best detoxifying herbs, vegetables, and fruits that are gentle enough to use during fasting:

- *Milk Thistle* is good for liver cleansing and support.
- *Dandelion* is an effective blood purifier and general organ cleanser.
- *Burdock Root* helps remove catabolic waste from cellular activity.

- *Slippery Elm* is very soothing to inflamed colon tissues and helps settle the stomach.
- *Yucca* is a natural anti-inflammatory, supports circulation, and reduces discomfort.
- *Garlic* is anti-bacterial, anti-viral, anti-fungal, and anti-parasitic.
- *Kombu* is a sea-vegetable that alkalizes the body and purifies the blood of fats.
- *Spirulina* is high in chlorophyll and aids enzyme production and digestion.
- *Carrots* are trace mineral-rich, high in vitamins, and alkalize the body.
- *Beets* provide several supportive nutrients, fiber, and flavor.
- *Parsnips* support detoxification of the kidneys.
- *Spinach* is an excellent source of nutrients and trace minerals.
- *Celery* is trace mineral-rich, high in vitamins, alkalizing, and flavorful to pets.
- *Parsley* is trace mineral-rich, oxygenating to the blood, and helps detoxify odors.
- *Ginger* can help the digestive system, reduces gas, and aids in reducing hypertension.
- *Apples* provide energy while supporting detoxification.
- *Cranberries* are very high in Vitamin C, help flush urinary tract waste.
- *Papaya* re-balances and aids digestion, and helps flush wastes.

Avoid highly acidic vegetables like tomatoes and onions (which can be deadly to dogs), or difficult-to-digest ingredients like cabbage. Also avoid the use of harsh fibers such as psyllium, which can further irritate and damage sensitive intestinal tissues. Although a good ingredient for producing bulk and encouraging elimination, psyllium's negative side effects outweigh its benefits during detoxification.

## HOMEOPATHIC DETOXIFICATION

Homeopathic detoxification encourages elimination and works well when combined with fasting, or used alone. One or several individual homeopathic remedies may be chosen, based on your pet's individual needs, or you may find that one of the many combination remedies available will work just as well. For detoxification it is best to work within the lower potencies, Xs to low Cs. Homeopathic detoxification should be used daily for no less than two weeks, preferably six to eight weeks. Give one daily dose at bedtime for most cases, or one dose upon rising and again at bedtime for more chronic cases.

Sometimes it is advisable to allow an initial build-up of the remedy by frequent dosing. Give one dose every fifteen minutes for the first hour (four times) when beginning detoxification and any other time you feel that your pet might need a little extra detoxifying boost. You cannot overdose your pet. Each repeated dose enhances the effect.

After the initial detoxification process, a maintenance program can be initiated on a weekly basis. One dose once a week at bedtime will help process current waste build-up, stimulate proper kidney and liver function, and support general good health. Do not use homeopathic detoxification in lieu of proper feeding, supplementing, and general care. It should be used to support biological functions such as digestion and elimination.

## HOMEOPATHIC REMEDIES FOR DETOXIFICATION

- *Antimonium Crudum* is good for gout-like symptoms with gastric weaknesses.
- *Arsenicum Album* is used for general detoxification, and to rebalance the liver and spleen.
- *Berberis Vulgaris* is good for a gouty constitution, particularly for a pet with a history of poor nutrition.

- *Bryonia* helps digestive problems that contribute to the accumulation of waste.
- *Cadium Sulph.* balances basic disease with gastric involvement.
- *Carduus Marianus* supports the vascular system, gall bladder, and liver.
- *Chelidonium Majus* is a liver remedy used for degenerative diseases.
- *Hydrastis* improves liver action and stimulates the immune system.
- *Juniperus Communis* encourages kidney elimination.
- *Solidago Vira* supports kidney detoxification.
- *Taraxacum* is used for bilious attacks and flatulence associated with cleansing.
- *Nux Vomica* helps to counter nausea, irritability, digestive disturbances, and portal congestion sometimes associated with the detoxification process.

*Nux Vomica* is often the first remedy homeopaths choose to establish equilibrium of biological functions and to counteract many chronic effects. It should always be included, regardless of what other remedies are chosen. The best homeopathic combinations for detoxification include this remedy. I have used *Arsenicum Album* and *Nux Vomica* to reverse many acute toxic reactions (including pesticide poisonings). When in doubt, this is a sound combination to try.

## WHAT TO EXPECT DURING DETOXIFICATION

Since detoxification removes waste from the body, waste will present itself during the detoxification process. Sometimes the symptoms you are trying to address with the cleansing process are aggravated. This is a good sign! Called a curative response, it is a clear indicator that the body has been stimulated into cleansing. Curative responses are a natural part of detoxification and are vital to strengthening and re-balancing the body. When this response occurs, the first impulse many people have is to run to the veterinarian to get a drug to suppress the resulting symptoms. Don't do it!

In striving to reach your pet's fullest curative potential, it is vital to the process that symptoms be *supported* rather than *suppressed*. More so than at any other time, suppression of these symptoms—even through the use of holistic animal care, rather than drugs—will only force the underlying imbalance deeper. The use of chemicals and medications—especially steroids and antibiotics—will also severely burden the body and the cleansing process.

Sometimes people will prematurely terminate the cleansing process because they fear the return or worsening of their pet's symptoms. Although symptoms may have been suppressed only through natural methods, if the cleansing process is terminated prematurely, you and your pet will eventually have to go through the process again if you desire true healing. It is best to address the symptoms gently (naturally), while continuing detoxification. Many things can be done to help minimize the aggravation (curative response) your pet experiences, without suppressing the cleansing and strengthening process. The safest, most effective way to support symptom aggravations is through the gentle modalities of nutritional supplements, homeopathy, flower essences, and herbs. (See "Symptoms A to Z" to address specific symptoms.)

Please note that aggravations do not have to occur for a successful detoxification. It is more common for the process to happen relatively easily, regardless of the pet's previous condition.

Pets who seemed to be healthy prior to detoxification can exhibit the worst symptoms, perhaps from an imbalance that was suppressed long ago. The bottom line is that you must be aware of your own pet's individual process and support that, regardless of any preconceived notions you may have had regarding what the process should be like. Each time the body experiences a curative response, which has been supported rather than suppressed, the body is strengthened, and the symptoms will return less frequently and less aggressively until eventually the symptoms are eliminated (reversed) completely.

Please, do not forget the power of love. Spend time nurturing your pet even if only to respect her or his need to be quiet and sleep more during this process of symptom reversal. Such tenderness will certainly help minimize any stress they may be experiencing.

## HINTS TO AID THE GENERAL DETOXIFICATION PROCESS

*Provide plenty of pure water.* Water is needed to help flush wastes as they are eliminated. Avoid using tap water containing chlorine and chemicals (which may be too harsh for the kidneys to handle), or distilled water which may facilitate too rapid a detoxification. Be sure that your pet's drinking water is always free of metals and sediments.

*Groom daily.* Grooming is necessary to brush away toxins that are being eliminated through the skin. Grooming also stimulates circulation, which increases elimination. Removal of old, dead skin also stimulates the growth of new, healthier coats. Wipe away any ear, eye, penile, vaginal, or anal discharges to avoid infections.

*Provide daily exercise in fresh air and sunshine.* This is necessary to encourage respiration, which supports the removal of deeper toxins. This also improves your pet's attitude, which supports healing. For indoor-only cats or small dogs, please provide a screened-in area where fresh air and sunshine can still be enjoyed.

*Respect your pet's quiet times.* Do so even if the pet's withdrawal from interaction with the family troubles you. It is normal for pets going through detoxification to sleep more, continue the fasting process on their own when they need to, become irritable, or seek out warmer or cooler areas.

*Avoid the use of all chemicals and drugs* that are not absolutely necessary for sustaining life. They will severely interfere in the detoxification process and may even be more harmful to your pet during this time. As the cleansing process moves deeper into the body, your pet's reaction to these substances may be stronger than before, and it is possible there may be an allergic reaction.

*Avoid giving a vaccine booster* within six weeks prior to, or after, a deep detoxification. The body may have more difficulty detoxifying shortly after a vaccination, or may react more strongly than usual. Excessive shedding is common.

*Address symptom aggravations gently* through the use of nutritional supplementation, homeopathy, flower essences, or herbs. This will allow the cleansing process to continue while keeping the symptoms from becoming too uncomfortable for your pet.

*Keep track of your pet's progress* to help you better understand the process. If you jot down a few notes each day, you will be less likely to scare yourself into thinking that it has been days since your pet last ate, when it isn't true.

If three days ago an abscess appeared and the discharge was clear but now has turned yellow, you will need to add natural antibiotics such as *garlic* or *Echinacea* to fight any infections that may have started. Keep track of how many days the discharge remains yellow or how quickly it responded to the supplements so that you may seek out other support if needed. On the other hand, if you notice that the abscess took two weeks to clear up, then returned in three weeks, only took four days to clear up that time, and did not return for two months the next time, you will begin to see a pattern that indicates you are on the right track.

## COMMON SYMPTOMS OF DETOXIFICATION

*Abscesses* can erupt during the detoxification process, especially around the chest and back. (See "Symptoms A to Z.")

*Dehydration* can occur when there is excessive vomiting or diarrhea, which causes an imbalance of nutrients and electrolytes. Dehydration will quickly shut down bodily functions and will reduce the effectiveness of the detoxification process. To check for dehydration in a cat or small dog, grab the skin from the back of the neck between your forefinger and thumb, pull it gently upwards, and release it. In medium- to large-sized dogs, you can also press the side of the lip up and release it. The skin in either case should snap back into place within a second or two. If it takes longer, then dehydration is a problem. If the skin doesn't snap back (this is very serious), consult your veterinarian immediately for subcutaneous fluid replacement therapy. In all other instances you can easily re-hydrate your pet by encouraging them to drink water or by using a syringe, free of its needle.

Provide one ounce of water per pound of body weight, per day. Electrolyte solutions can be added to the water if the animal seems weakened by the dehydration.

*Diarrhea* can sometimes occur, especially as old fecal materials are processed, or as a side effect of general detoxification. One or two doses daily of homeopathic *Arsenicum* and *Nux Vomica*, helpful when nausea is also present, will generally firm up the stool while continuing to support elimination. If the diarrhea is severe or very watery, use this remedy more frequently, every fifteen minutes for the first hour and then every hour afterward, until the diarrhea is resolved. *Slippery Elm* is a soothing herb for the colon during and after a bout with diarrhea. In this case, use powdered *Slippery Elm* instead of the extract or tincture. To be certain that your animal is not dehydrating, due to the loss of fluids through the diarrhea, watch how much water your pet drinks and check for the physical signs.

*Discharges* from all orifices are normal during detoxification. These are the routes that toxins can take directly out of the body. If your pet has a history of skin, ear, or eye irritations, nasal discharges, impacted anal glands (blocked discharge), mucous-coated stools, etc., you can expect an aggravation of these symptoms. Keep these areas clean, and utilize homeopathic remedies. *Arsenicum* is helpful as a general remedy, or you may want to explore others more directly suited to your pet's symptoms. No matter where these discharges originate, *Calcarea Carbonica* is an excellent constitutional remedy for watery to thicker discharges, and *Pulsatilla* is suited for discharges that are thick and yellow to greenish in color.

*Dry, flaky skin* can be easily cared for with a good brushing, terry cloth rub, and the application of some *Jojoba* or *Tea Tree* oil conditioner. Flaking of old skin cells is a normal part of detoxification, as old tissue is replaced by healthier skin. One or two doses of homeopathic *Sulphur* can also be very beneficial at this time. *M.S.M.* is a nutritional sulfur supplement that helps tissue repair and growth. The herb *Horsetail* also contains a high concentration of naturally occurring sulfur.

Frequent bathing can rob the skin of necessary oils causing an excessive release of these oils, which is the body's attempt to rebalance the skin. Avoid bathing your pet more often than every few weeks.

*Fever* can be a good sign during detoxification, as long as the overall condition of the animal is stable. If your pet appears to be severely exhausted, you may need to call a veterinarian. Fever supports detoxification, indicating that the body's defenses are working to burn up toxins, and old viral or bacterial infections. If you suspect a fever after twenty-four hours of fasting or a few weeks of ongoing detoxification and dietary improvements, realize that it is a normal part of the detoxification process. However, support is needed to keep the fever from weakening the body. Homeopathic remedies work best in this case. I recommend that you use *Phosphorus* for fever. If the fever is the result of an infection, increase garlic supplements, and add herbal products such as *Standardized Grapefruit Extract*, *Astragalus Root*, *Echinacea*, or *Golden Seal Root*, all excellent, safe natural antibiotics. If the fever is high, especially with debilitating side effects and lasts more than two days, seek veterinary advice.

*Flatulence* can be a problem during cleansing, because old fecal material is being eliminated. Detoxification increases peristalsis (the muscular contractions of the colon, which move fecal matter along and help to break it down). It's like turning over a well-decomposed compost heap so that the decayed material can be exposed and the odors released into the air. A good dose of *Arsenicum* and *Nux Vomica* will also help relieve flatulence.

*Infections* respond well to herbal support. Increase garlic supplementation and add *Standardized Grapefruit Extract* (I highly recommend Nutri-Biotic's *Citracidal*), *Echinacea*, and/or *Golden Seal Root*. These are all excellent, safe, and very effective natural antibiotics, which will work on the source of the infection and stimulate the immune system as well.

A homeopathic remedy that promotes drainage or a combination of remedies for infections can also be supportive in stimulating the body's defenses against the infection. Remedies that work well include *Antimonium Crudum* for skin infections with oozing and thick, yellow crusts, *Kal. Mur*. and *Kal. Phos.* (two types of tissue cell salts that aid in infections) or *Bioplasma* (the combination of all twelve tissue cell salts), and *Arsenicum*.

*Loss of appetite.* First determine if there is any fever present. Feed up to 100 mg. of *B-Complex vitamins* per day for cats or dogs. Many multiple vitamin/mineral products already include B vitamins, so check to see what you are already giving your pet first. A few doses of *Arsenicum* (in general), *Nux Vomica* (if accompanied by one or more symptoms including nausea, vomiting, stool problems, or flatulence) or *Belladonna* (if accompanied by nausea, empty retching and vomiting, as well as an aversion to drinking) should be used. A dose or two daily, especially fifteen minutes prior to feeding, can also help stimulate appetite. Several flower essences, especially a combination formulation for minimizing stress, can often settle an animal enough so that it begins to regain some appetite. Always address emotional stress when appetite loss is evident, as it can often be a contributing factor.

*Skin eruptions* are the most common of detoxification symptoms. *Horsetail* and *Milk Thistle* are excellent herbs to use at this time, but homeopathic remedies such as *Apis* or *Sepia* (dry, rashly skin), *Rhus Tox.* (for clusters of tiny pimples that are extremely itchy), or *Graphites* (for scabby, oozy eruptions) work quickly to relieve irritation and discomfort. When in doubt try a dose of *Arsenicum* or *Sulphur*, both general skin remedies. *Antimonium Crudum* is best with staphylococcal or streptococcal infections, but follow the recommendations for infections as well.

*Vomiting* can also lead to dehydration and is often a symptom of detoxification, rather than an attempt to rid the stomach of an irritant. Since persistent vomiting will quickly exhaust your pet, it is best to suppress this symptom quickly. Homeopathy works well, and is easier to administer, because it won't trigger vomiting like an herb would. For vomiting after eating, a combination of *Arsenicum* and *Nux Vomica* is effective. When vomiting occurs after drinking, use *Phosphorus* (with or without *Arsenicum*). Give one dose of each, every fifteen minutes for the first hour, then one dose every hour, until there has been no more vomiting for one hour. (See "Symptoms A to Z.")

## PROPER NUTRITION

The primary line of defense to prevent or treat skin and coat conditions is a sound nutritional program. After detoxification is an ideal time to introduce a healthier diet.

Your pet's natural diet should consist of fresh, high-quality, easy to digest and assimilate ingredients. Since home cooking is optimal, but not very practical for many people, you should seek a quality commercial product. Become an educated label reader, look beyond catchy terms such as "natural," "organic," "skin conditioning," "allergy diet," and "human-grade quality," and ask the manufacturer directly to prove the quality of their products and guarantee their formula.

Seek only Grade A or B meats (human grade) and avoid the four-D meats—dead, dying, diseased, or disabled animals not fit for human consumption. Four-D meats are those most commonly used in pet foods.

Grain by-products are prevalent, problematic ingredients in many commercial pet products. These include wheat millings, brewer's rice (waste from brewing), and flours. These inexpensive fillers are not only devoid of nutritional value, but can also severely compromise your pet's health. Manufacturers often include rancid and moldy grains in their products because they are inexpensive. These poor-quality grain by-products increase the possibility of a toxic reaction. Only Grade 1 or 2 grains (human grades) should be used, preferably whole ground, to ensure that their nutritional goodness remains intact.

People are often concerned that changing their pet's diet will only result in digestive upsets. This is true only if you are changing from a poor-quality or chemical-based diet to another one of the same quality. When you switch to a healthier, more natural diet, there should be no irritating ingredients to upset the balance. The only problems your pet might experience are soft stool and gas. This can happen because you may be overfeeding your pet with the new diet.

One cup of a grocery store food is almost fifty percent filler! A better brand of grocery-type foods, even pet shop pet food or prescription diets, can be just as bad. These may have less filler, but they will probably contain other types of by-products, which may alter the quantity of nutrients available in one cup. When switching to a higher-quality food, there generally is less filler, and, therefore, feeding the same quantities (cup for cup) would result in overfeeding of the better brand. Carefully read and follow the manufacturer's recommendations for the food, and watch your pet carefully for the first few weeks to see how they react.

Overfeeding can often occur when people begin to cook for their pets. It is difficult to recommend one recipe that will suit everybody's needs, so I suggest that you seek out a well-researched book on natural pet care that includes recipes.

Beware of feeding your pet raw meats, which can upset, rather than support your pet's condition. I believe this is because animals adapt to fit their environment. Our pets have been domesticated for so long that they have been altered to become processed food eaters and have lost the wild animal's ability to digest raw meat tissue, bone, hide, feathers, etc., on a regular basis. Even if you give your pet a digestive enzyme, your pet will probably have to struggle to digest raw animal tissue.

If you prefer home-cooked foods to commercially processed pet foods, and you will lightly cook the food so that all the enzymes and nutrients are not destroyed, cooking will break down the meat sufficiently, making it easier for your pet's digestive tract to handle.

Even with the best-quality and balanced diet (cooked or home-cooked), nutritional supplementation is necessary to provide many nutrients now missing from our food chain. For instance, research indicates that fifty years ago spinach had up to eighty percent more nutritional value than it does today. This is true in varying degrees for other vegetables, grains, and fruits, as well as meats from animals fed "off the land." Our earth has been stripped of many of the naturally occurring micronutrients found in soil, which are then assimilated by plants. Years of over-farming, toxic chemical or fertilizer use, and environmental pollution (such as acid rain) have taken their toll.

Even organic farming methods can not guarantee that the produce is more nutritious, as it will take organic farmers approximately seventy-five years of organic farming before these nutrients are returned to the soil. Therefore, it is important that we supplement our animals' diets to ensure that they receive the fundamental nutrients required. Pet foods which are "nutritionally complete" according to AAFCO (American Association of Feed Control Officers) still may not provide all that is needed for basic good health. For instance, the AAFCO standards require a certain amount of protein per cup of food, but that protein does not have to be digestible. So what good is it? This is also true for certain sources of Vitamin A or calcium, among other nutrients.

Proper nutrition not only includes quality, easy to digest foods, but also appropriate supplementation to support health. Such a regime will stimulate your pet's curative potential, and also increase that ability to reverse any adverse symptom.

## KEY INGREDIENTS FOR A HEALTHY DIET

- *Fresh ingredients* that do not have an unpleasant odor due to rancidity
- *Whole foods* such as whole ground grains, not "flours," "mill runs," or "by-products"
- *Concentrated protein sources known* as "meal" (as in "lamb meal" or "beef meal") is preferred over whole meats (listed only as "lamb"). This is not to be confused with "by-product meal."

"Meal" simply refers to the process of removing up to eighty percent, but no less than forty-five percent, of the ingredient's water content. There is more meat protein for your money, since water only adds to the weight of the ingredients. Weight is listed on the product label by the heaviest to lightest ingredient. It is very deceiving to find chicken, (or turkey, rabbit, fish, and other animal sources) listed first, when the majority of protein is coming from grains, not animal protein. The cost of the product is considerably less when a protein other than an animal protein is used. One pound of meal is equal to approximately three pounds of whole meat, and since there is an additional charge to dehydrate it , many companies use the meat to draw you to the label, but use a cheaper ingredient for the actual protein—a protein source that could trigger symptoms.

Look for *identifiable and digestible animal protein* or *fat sources* such as beef, beef meal, lamb, lamb meal, lamb fat, chicken, chicken meal or chicken fats, turkey, ostrich, etc., not vague terms like "meats," "mammal," or "animal fats."

Look for *USDA Grade A or B animal protein sources*, preferably raised without growth hormones or recently given antibiotics.

Look for *USDA Grade 1 or 2 whole grains*, preferably free of chemical pesticides or herbicides. Organic grains are not cost-effective for use in commercial pet foods yet (if your pet's food claims "organic," demand written certification), but "pesticide-free" or "washed grains" are available. Beans are an excellent source of protein as well. If you are cooking for your pet at home, buy the best you can afford.

*Balanced, combined proteins and grain sources* suit most pets better than single source ingredients, contrary to popular belief. Vegetable and fruit fiber should be present, such as carrots and apples, for proper digestion, natural flavoring, and trace nutrients. Fiber is important to elimination and is nutrient-rich. Quality sources of fat are necessary for energy and good coats. Vegetable or fish oils should be used, rather than animal fats. Because cats have a higher metabolism than dogs, they need the higher fat content, and high-quality animal fats are acceptable.

*Price*. Often, the cheaper foods are actually more expensive, meal for meal, because you have to feed so much more than a better-quality diet, with less filler.

*Product should be fresh when purchased.* Check the manufacture date, not the expiration date. Manufacturers will never admit the food won't really last a year. Never feed your pet food, especially naturally preserved food, that is older than six months, unless it has a completely sealed, airtight, barrier bag. Stale food not only doesn't taste good, it has lost most of its nutritional value through oxidation, and the ingredients are no longer as bio-available.

## INGREDIENTS TO AVOID IN A HEALTHY DIET

*Foul-smelling ingredients* should be avoided at all costs. No matter what the date is on the bag, smell it when you open the bag and, if it smells rancid, don't feed it to your pet.

*Greasy food.* If you see oil on the bag or feel a sticky residue on cans of pet food, it is high in animal fats or tallow. These can include rendered carcasses and recycled cooking grease from restaurants. These fats are difficult to digest and often rancid prior to the manufacturing process.

*Animal by-products* such as "beef by-product," "lamb by-product," and "chicken by-product" are a mixture of the whole carcass including feces, cancerous tumors, hide, hooves, beaks, feathers, and fur. "Meat" or "meat by-products" are a mixture of whatever mammals, including road kill, rats, and other dogs and cats ground together. Avoid "fish by-product" and especially "poultry by-products," which are a mixture of whatever feathered animals, including pigeons, ground together and should definitely not be fed to your pet.

*Grain by-products* such as "mill runs," "flours," "middlings," "husks," and "parts" should be avoided. They have no nutritional value because all the available nutrients have been removed. They may be harsh to an animal's digestive and eliminatory tracts, and irritate the body as it attempts to process them. These cheap fillers are used as additional protein sources to increase the finished product's weight and mass, although they are non-digestible and therefore cannot be assimilated.

*Fillers* such as powdered "cellulose" and "cellulose fiber" can include recycled newspaper, sawdust, and cardboard. "Plant cellulose" is usually ground peanut hulls—which are very damaging to sensitive colon tissues. Beet pulp or grain by-products have no significant nutritional value, but do add bulk and weight to the finished product.

*Yeast* is a cheap source of B vitamins, amino acids, and some nutrients. Touted for flea control and a shiny coat, yeast can contribute to poor skin and coat conditions by burdening the liver and interfering with proper digestion.

*Sugar* is added to most commercial diets and treats. On pet food labels it can be called "sucrose," "beet pulp," "molasses," "cane syrup," "fruit solids," and of course, "sugar." It is a very cheap, heavy filler (cost effective for the manufacturer) and is also addictive (the pet will want more of the same). Additional sugar in the diet is the primary trigger of excessive shedding, weight problems, diabetic conditions, and behavioral problems in pets.

# Symptom Reversal

Once you have established a good foundation by detoxification and proper diet so that the body can draw strength to fuel its curative process, it is time to address the individual needs of your pet. Although the basic curative process is the same for all living beings, each one of us has our own unique journey toward symptom reversal.

All of our symptoms have a history, unique to our own experiences. A youthful body can handle a multitude of stresses and maintain some balance. As the body grows older and its biological processes slow down, the body can become overwhelmed by its lifestyle.

Your pet's age, how genetically compromised he or she is, the quality of his or her lifestyle, and the severity and duration of the symptoms determine the history of disease and the curative process. I have never seen an animal that was too old, too weak, too young, too sick, or too hopeless to respond to holistic animal care. Is every case a complete success? That depends on your definition of success. Every animal's symptoms, when addressed holistically, experienced some positive change.

Seventy-five percent of pets respond immediately to detoxification and nutritional support, and a large number experience long-term symptom reversal. Fifteen percent need additional naturopathic (including acupuncture or acupressure, chiropractic, and massage), plus homeopathic and/or herbal support, to complete the curative process and effectively reverse their skin and coat conditions.

Eight percent of pets might need some medical or chemical support: short-term symptom suppression through antihistamines or antibiotics (when symptoms are severely damaging to the pet's overall health) and steroids (when lack of curative response is life threatening). Many severely compromised animals can benefit from short-term support until the natural support they are receiving takes over. Unfortunately, about half of these animals were given chemicals because the body's attempts to rebalance were misunderstood. Classic symptoms of detoxification were visible, but the owner or veterinarian arrested the process with medical treatment. Some of these owners later used detoxification procedures successfully, but others remained in the cycle of symptom suppression for years before they allowed the detoxification process to be completed. Others simply gave up.

Two percent of suffering pets will always have poor skin and coat condition, slow tissue healing, and/or chronic infection no matter how we care for them. Symptoms can be suppressed holistically and/or chemically for short-term relief, but as soon as treatment is stopped, the cycle begins anew. These pets are either too genetically compromised or too overwhelmed by their condition to ever successfully reverse their disease on their own. Remember that the more holistic the lifestyle, the easier it will be for your pet to resist toxins, and for their biological functions to remain healthy—even if you choose to use medications along with holistic practices. Each year your pet lives a holistic lifestyle, his or her body will continue to strengthen, many symptoms will become easier to address, or may reverse themselves with time. Detoxification also protects the liver, kidneys, and other vital organs from toxic drug side effects.

Common sense is your most valuable tool to reverse symptoms. Ask yourself if what you are doing is getting you the results you want. If not, re-evaluate, but do continue addressing the problem in the same way. Not doing something is *not* an option. *Nothing comes from nothing.* People often exclaim, "I thought I'd just wait and see if it got any better on its own." They are shocked that the condition gets worse! By the time they do something, it can be too late. The body may be too weakened, or the disease may be too deep, and it becomes so much harder to regain balance!

The only time that it is appropriate to *do* nothing is during detoxification or a curative response, during which time the health of the animal may temporarily become worse as the body attempts to rebalance itself. To do something (to suppress) during this time only stops the process, and drives the imbalance deeper into the body.

It is appropriate to address symptoms through holistic animal care when:

- Any non-life-threatening symptom has been present for four to eight hours.
- There are acute (sudden) symptoms from overexertion or toxins: rashes, pustules, digestive upset, discharges, stiffness, irritability or emotional stress, including withdrawal (often the results of exhaustion due to excessive scratching or pain).
- There are acute flare-ups of chronic (ongoing) symptoms, especially during detoxification.
- Known triggers are present, such as during high-exposure days. Many of my symptom reversal suggestions can also be applied as a preventative.
- A curative response has been ongoing for more than forty-eight hours.

It is appropriate to address symptoms through allopathic, veterinary care when:

- There exists any life-threatening acute symptom, especially paralysis, respiratory difficulties resulting in hyper-panting, an excessive heart rate present for two to four hours, loss of consciousness, excessive dehydration, or uncontrollable shaking.
- High fever is present for more than twenty-four hours.
- Chronic symptom aggravation for more than twenty-four hours results in loss of mobility, uncontrollable digestive upsets, urinary dysfunction, or other severe symptoms.

- Unmanageable infectious states, *even if mild*, have lasted for four to six weeks.

When in doubt, seek out a trusted professional to support your pet's process.

## HELPFUL HINTS

*Feed a high-quality diet and supplement at least twice per day*—more often if needed to help stabilize blood sugar, support the immune system, and reduce the toxic load.

*Supplement with the proper nutrients*, including glandular products and herbs, for a strong foundation from which to stimulate the body's curative response.

*Utilize homeopathy* to help maximize the body's curative potential, especially the processes of detoxification and symptom reversal.

*Use synergistic modalities* such as chiropractic care, massage, touch and energy therapies including giving acupressure therapy at home in-between veterinary acupuncture sessions. Home therapy will prolong the benefits received in a clinical visit.

*Maintain a holistic animal care lifestyle*, even in-between cycles of symptoms, to help enhance the body's defenses and further balance the body's weaknesses. With each month the body will gain balance and strength, including immune support and resistance to general sensitivities. Remember, symptom suppression—even holistically *but* without constitutional support—only leads to a reoccurrence of symptoms, not a long-term reversal of disease.

*Do not underestimate the power of nature;* recognize that nature can take longer to suppress a symptom than a drug, but often will do the job more completely.

*Support the curative power of nature* and avoid interfering with it. Use chemicals and medications carefully. Avoid vaccinations whenever possible.

*Use common sense.* Address changes in your animal's health or behavior as soon as possible, pay attention to what your pet's symptoms are telling you. For example, if your dog's skin irritation and shedding increases the day after a bath, don't keep using the same shampoo or bathe him so frequently.

*Don't sabotage the healing process* by incorrectly utilizing diets, veterinarian-prescribed medications, or natural supplement products. Read the directions. Ask questions! The more you know and understand, the more successful you will be.

Remember, it can take three to six weeks for detoxification and increased assimilation of nutrients to begin establishing the necessary foundation for a successful curative process. During this time old cells are replaced with newer, healthier skin and coat cells, which will bring change to the overall condition. Therefore, it is best to allow the body some time to respond on its own before adding too many ingredients to the mix. Provide a high-quality multiple vitamin and mineral supplement with basic herbal or homeopathic support for the first month or two, until you better understand the specific underlying imbalance. Remember that nearly eight out of ten pets successfully reverse their symptoms with this alone. Additional supplements or medications may overwhelm the body with ingredients it doesn't need and interfere with the body's natural healing ability. Carefully research each product available to see what is specifically recommended in your situation. Be sure to read ingredient labels carefully, and follow all instructions listed on any products you choose to use on your animals.

Homeopathy is safe to use in addition to herbs or medications, although allopathic drugs may interfere with a homeopathic remedy's potential to activate the curative process. Homeopathy can aid in the reduction of acute flare-ups and supports symptom reversal on a deeper level than either herbs or supplements alone. Homeopathic remedies often can be the keys to reversing a deeper acute or chronic weakness. To use homeopathic remedies to their fullest potential, follow a few simple suggestions. Although a lot of emphasis is placed on potencies, I have found many remedies to be successful in a wide range of potencies. I suggest that you use whatever potency is available whether it is a 6X or a 3C. For the majority of acute reactions, even if due to chronic conditions, utilizing the lower potencies will effect change. These potencies range anywhere from 3X to 30C. For long-term reversal of a specific disorder, utilizing the higher 200C potency will be effective after lower potencies have brought the acute reaction under control. High potencies, such as Ms, should be used under professional guidance. By giving the body a boost with homeopathic remedies, other supplements act more quickly and effectively.

When beginning a homeopathic remedy, build up its action in the body through frequent dosing. You cannot overdose your pet. Give one dose orally, according to the manufacturer's recommendations, every fifteen minutes for the first hour, then once every hour until there is relief. To maintain relief, dose a minimum of twice daily for an additional week or two. More frequent dosing may be administered as needed. Resume homeopathic treatment or any another appropriate remedy whenever the symptom presents itself, and follow this schedule until there is complete reversal. Long-term maintenance is also possible through a weekly dose of the most beneficial remedy.

I prefer liquid remedies because they are easier to administer. If the dropper touches your hands or your pet, rinse it off before returning it to the bottle. Most remedies come in sugar pellets (use as is) or tablets (crush inside a piece of paper first for best application). To avoid contamination and a reduction in efficacy, do not handle these remedies with your bare hands. Rather, use the cap or a clean piece of paper to administer the dose. Always give homeopathic remedies at least fifteen minutes before or after meals and at least fifteen minutes before or after the administration of strong therapeutic extracts.

# Symptoms A to Z

This chapter lists the most common symptoms associated with skin and coat problems, as well as some that are more commonly associated with allergies, but which create related symptoms. Your pet may be experiencing a slightly different symptom than described here. Please try to match your particular needs as closely as possible to one of the symptoms listed.

**Abscesses** can erupt especially around the chest and back. This occurs most frequently during a curative response or detoxification process. As one of its defenses against toxins, the body will pocket an irritating substance or allergen (sometimes for years) to keep it from establishing a deeper hold on the body. Detoxification releases these toxins from the fatty tissue where they are stored and releases them into the bloodstream for elimination. Since the skin is the largest eliminatory organ, abscesses may occur. At the first sign of swelling and accompanying heat, a dose of homeopathic *Belladonna* or *Sulphur* may discourage the full formation of an abscess.

Whether you suspect a foreign object or not, use the homeopathic remedy *Silica*, which encourages eruption and drainage. Since the abscess itself is a foreign object, *Silica* will generally work well. If not, try *Mercurius*, especially if thick pus has formed and the surrounding skin has become angrier. Apply a warm, damp cloth to the area for fifteen minutes at a time to encourage eruption of the abscess. This will also soothe your pet. Homeopathic *Hepar Sulphuricum* is the best remedy for abscesses too painful to touch. It can be used in conjunction with the *Silica*.

Once there is drainage, be sure to keep the area clean and dry. It is helpful to trim away a little fur around the site to expose it to more air. This encourages healing and makes it easier to treat the abscess topically. Clean it with a solution of fifty-percent hydrogen peroxide and fifty-percent water, then apply a little *Tea Tree or Calendula lotion* to encourage healing and prevent worse infections. Treat topically at least once a day, twice a day if the abscess is large and angry. (See Infections.)

**Adrenal Malfunction** is common in animals who also exhibit allergic reactions, especially those with chronic skin conditions. Often, it can be caused by previous cycles of steroid treatments, which are commonly used to suppress allergy-related symptoms. You may want to recommend a book to your veterinarian entitled *Pet Allergies: Remedies for an Epidemic*, by Alfred J. Plechner, DVM, and Martin Zucker.

Testing for hormonal or cortisol levels is beneficial, no matter what you decide to do. If nothing has seemed to work, utilize any medication that is appropriate for you and your animal. Pets who have not responded well to natural modalities are often diagnosed with deeper glandular malfunctions, which, when addressed, help stimulate the curative process.

There are many excellent natural glandular products available. I prefer *glandulars in powder or tablet form* to homeopathic ones, but do not disregard a homeopathic remedy combined with a potentized glandular *in addition to* a tableted form. Homeopathic glandulars work on a deeper level and provide overall support, whereas tableted glandulars feed the gland directly, providing more substantial support in reversing glandular weakness. *Multi-glandulars*, a combination of several glands, are beneficial in supporting the weaker gland, but make sure the combination you use contains sufficient amounts of the particular gland you need to stimulate and support. Add another single glandular product to the multiple, if needed. (See Cushing's Disease.)

**Aggression** can be a problem in pets suffering from sensitivies or chronic skin problems. More commonly the ingredients in pet products themselves, especially sugars and chemical preservatives, contribute to the toxins and skin reaction, and trigger the aggression as well. In addition, some animals cannot tolerate the constant itching and irritation caused by skin irritations and shedding. They exhaust themselves from scratching or biting and lash out when approached.

Avoid stress, sudden movements, and abrupt awakening of your pet, factors that tend to trigger an outburst. Be sure that you are using *higher potencies of Vitamin B1, B2, B6:* 50 mg. to 100 mg. for cats and dogs regardless of size and *B12:* 50 mcg. to 125 mcg. for cats and dogs. Also use homeopathic *Aconite* for sudden or intense fear, or *Ignatia* for grief and anger. *Bryonia* is helpful when the slightest movement seems painful to your pet, and the aggression may be based in part to a pain response. Several flower essences, such as *Chicory, Holly, Impatiens, Rock Rose,* and *Vine* can also be helpful, as well as additional exercise. Many aggressive pets have noticeable improvements in their dispositions shortly after the detoxification process.

**Allergy Reactions** in general can be successfully suppressed with a few doses of homeopathy in lower potencies (3X to 30C). Give one dose orally, according to the manufacturer's recommendations, every fifteen minutes for the first hour, then every hour until there is relief. Give homeopathic remedies at least fifteen minutes before or after food or strong extracts. Treat the most obvious symptom first, and then focus on any specific symptoms next.

### *Homeopathic Remedies for Allergic Reactions*

- *Arsenicum* is used for general irritations, hot spots, digestive imbalances, or toxicity-related symptoms such as reactive arthritis.
- *Sulphur* is used for a wide variety of skin conditions associated with intense itching, which becomes worse at night in warm surroundings. Scratching may seem to satisfy the pet temporarily, but often will result in increased itching and burning. *Sulphur* is also good for greasy skin.
- *Apis* is good for intensely itchy skin that is aggravated by warmth, including the warmth the body may give off when covered in rashes.
- *Rhus Tox* is helpful when the animal is rubbing or scratching his or her skin, when the animal gets wet, or when cold weather seems to aggravate itchy skin. It is especially good for irritations about the head and reactive arthritis.
- *Urtica Urens* addresses extensive eruptions, hives, or welts that are very itchy. Usually the skin is dry and aggravated by warmth or bathing. (These conditions do not respond to *Apis* or *Sulphur*.) It is also good for profuse discharges from mucous membranes. Symptoms may be localized to the right side of the body.
- *Sabadilla* is a popular hay-fever remedy, addressing common upper-respiratory symptoms such as asthma, spasmodic sneezing, watery nasal discharge, facial itching, irritated ears, and red, runny eyes.
- *Euphrasia* is another excellent remedy for allergy-related eye and tear duct irritations.
- *Nux Vomica* addresses the majority of digestive imbalances, including gas, vomiting, diarrhea, or lack of appetite, especially when dosed with *Arsenicum*.

Herbal antihistamines and anti-inflammatory products are very effective and a good alternative to over-the-counter drugs, such as *Benadryl*, or veterinary prescriptions, such as *Prednisone*. I recommend that you use a combination of homeopathic remedies for acute reaction and herbs to lessen sensitivity, which may reduce a more severe reaction.

### *Herbs for Allergic Reactions*

- *Yucca Root* has been used for centuries by indigenous cultures to reduce general inflammation. Current studies have confirmed that bio-available steroidal saponins (found mostly in pure extract form, rather than the fibrous powder that is a waste product of extraction) perform as effectively as their chemical counterparts (steroids such as *Prednisone*), without the serious drug side effects. *Yucca* enhances the action of other, more specific-use herbs, in working more effectively by supporting liver function and detoxification.
- *Chinese Ephedra* is a powerful antihistamine, which quickly reduces inflammation. This herb has been abused as a stimulant, but it is very safe when used as directed. *Ephedra* reduces the itching of a histamine reaction and can be used for both topical (eyes, ears, skin) and internal (irritable bowels, inflamed respiratory passages) symptoms.
- *Marshmallow* and/or *Bayberry Root* reduces inflammation in general, and is helpful in histamine detoxification and in the reduction of respiratory stress.
- *Eyebright Herb* helps address general allergy symptoms affecting the eyes.
- *Stinging Nettle Leaf* reduces general redness and irritation of the skin, eyes, and ears. It can also help reduce irritation of the anal glands and inflamed joints.
- *Red Clover Blossoms* are useful in reversing skin eruptions, as well as reducing coughs and bronchitis. This herb supports immune function.
- *Eyebright*, *Bayberry Root Bark*, *Golden Seal Root*, *Calamus*, and *Stinging Nettle Leaf* act together to contract swollen mucous membranes associated with hay fever and allergies. The antibacterial properties of this combination help keep chronic infections of the eyes, ears, and respiratory system in check.
- *Turmeric Root*, *Black Catechu*, *Grindelia Floral Buds*, and *Lobelia*, combined, protect the liver from circulating antigens and allergens, thereby reducing infections and skin or intestinal irritations associated with airborne, urea, and food-related allergies. This combination provides support for the adrenal glands during epinephrine (adrenaline) excretion. Epinephrine is produced

by the body during inflammatory responses generated by allergens. This combination is also indicated for all disorders of hypersensitivity, including excessive shedding, allergies, dermatitis, irritable bowel syndrome, reactive arthritis, and food-related digestive disorders.

- *Red Clover Blossoms*, *Stinging Nettle Leaf*, *Cleavers Herb*, *Yellow Dock Root*, *Burdock Root*, *Yarrow Flowers*, *Plantain Leaf and Corm*, *Licorice Root*, and *Prickly Ash Bark* purify the blood and drain excess lymphatic fluids. This combination improves metabolism by carrying more blood and nutrients to the cells and thereby promoting greater excretion at the cellular level. It is useful for eczema, psoriasis, tumors, cysts, acne, excessive shedding, and other skin disorders such as mange. It is also helpful for lymphatic edema and toxemia, including reactive joint inflammation.

**Anal Glands** can become impacted in pets, especially dogs, who have been fed poor-quality diets and whose digestive and eliminatory systems do not function properly. Impacted anal glands cause irritation and itching around the anus. Pets will scoot their rear ends across the floor and chew at them, eventually infecting the area.

If the pet owner squeezes or drains these glands incorrectly, it will only damage them further, making them even more susceptible to impacting. Please have these glands professionally expressed by a veterinarian, no more than every six weeks at first, then tapering off until you can go yearly if needed.

You can encourage drainage of these glands by holding a compress, soaked in a warm solution of six ounces *pure water*, two ounces *Witch Hazel*, with twenty drops of *Calendula Extract*, ten drops of *Golden Seal Extract* and ten drops of *Yucca Extract*. Rinse well with a fresh solution, followed by a topical application of *Calendula*, *Tea Tree Oil*, and/or *Aloe Gel*. Keep some topical solution in the refrigerator; it will feel especially soothing on irritated and inflamed tissues.

Soak a cotton pad and hold it gently against the area for a few minutes, or spray it on as needed. Repeat twice to three times a day until swelling and redness is gone.

Apply *Vitamin E* and/or *Jojoba Oil* directly to tough or scared tissue to soften it. Avoid petroleum-based products, which will further irritate the area, and encourage bacterial infection. Such products can become poisonous if ingested frequently by your pet.

A few doses of *Apis* or *Hypericum* for irritation and *Arsenicum* or *Nux Vomica* for detoxification can greatly reduce discomfort. *Hepar Sulph* can help reverse infected glands. It is more effective when combined with *Arsenicum* or *Nux Vomica* and an herbal antibiotic such as *Echinacea* or *Golden Seal.*

Dried *Chinese mushrooms*, such as *Shiitake* and *Reishi*, are very healing to anal gland tissues, and together with other fiber-producing ingredients (apple pectin, guar gum, psyllium) can help stimulate a complete evacuation of stool from the colon, which will reduce toxic waste from backing up the anal glands. *Astragalus Root* is useful for prolapsed conditions of the anus and impacted anal glands. It works as a diuretic to flush wastes, reduce edema, and promote the discharge of pus. *Garlic* is also indicated. Don't forget flower remedies, such as *Mimulus*, or a *Rescue* combination, if your pet refuses to allow you near without a fight. (See Abscesses, Infections.)

**Anemia** is a common symptom associated with poor coat condition and color. I believe that many cases of anemia are the result of liver complications. Common side effects of anemia include lack of stamina, a depressed appetite, slow tissue repair, poor immune function, muscle weakness, pale-colored gums (including loss of mouth color), and dull eyes. Sometimes the faint odor of metal is present on the breath. More serious anemia needs proper diagnosis and treatment, but borderline anemia is commonly reversed with proper nutrition.

Anemia is the body's inability to produce more red blood cells to counteract the discarding of cells by the liver when this valuable organ becomes burdened, and begins to malfunction. Iron supplementation is a well-known treatment for anemia and will quickly reverse symptoms. Always use a good quality iron source such as an *iron proteinate*, which is a form of iron that is chelated with an amino acid for better absorption. Be careful not to over-supplement with iron, since iron can easily become toxic. The first symptom of toxicity is constipation. Limit daily levels to around 10 mg. for cats and small dogs, and 20 mg. for medium to large dogs. In addition, provide *chromium* to aid in iron assimilation. Chromium reduces the body's need for higher levels of iron. Also use *Alfalfa*; both in herbal (nutrient-rich) and in lower potency homeopathic form. *Taraxacum* is also a good homeopathic choice as is its herbal twin, *Dandelion*.

Although liver is a popular remedy for anemia, avoid feeding it on a regular basis. Liver is a primary detoxifying organ and stores excess toxins eliminated from the blood. When you feed this organ to your pet, you are also feeding concentrated toxins, including growth hormones and antibiotics.

**Appetite Problems**, especially loss of appetite, can occur during curative responses to disease. Appetite loss can also result from toxicity to drugs, especially antibiotics commonly prescribed for chronic skin complaints. Before you utilize holistic support for appetite loss, be sure there is no fever present and that your pet is not dehydrated. This is a more serious problem. (See Fever and Infection.) Also determine the level of stress your pet may be experiencing and address that, as stress can also interfere with appetite. (See

Behavioral Problems.)

For nutritional support, feed up to 100 mg. of B-Complex vitamins per day. This, in addition to a short fast, can quickly stimulate the appetite. Often, a lack of appetite is the result of a systemic toxic overload.

Try a few doses of *Arsenicum* for general appetite loss, *Nux Vomica* when appetite loss is accompanied by one or more symptoms including nausea, vomiting, stool problems, flatulence, or *Belladonna* when there is nausea, empty retching, and vomiting as well as an aversion to drinking. A dose or two daily, *especially 15 minutes prior to feeding*, can also help stimulate appetite. Several flower essences, especially *Mimulus*, *Star of Bethlehem*, and *Rock Rose*, or a combination, can often settle an animal enough so that it begins to regain an appetite.

**Behavioral Problems** are often associated with chronic skin irritations. (See Aggression.) Discomfort can trigger aggression, though some animals respond with nervousness, shyness, or complete withdrawal. Flower essences and homeopathic remedies work well to address the underlying emotional aspect of most behavioral problems.

***Flower Essences and Homeopathic Remedies for Behavioral Problems***

- *Star of Bethlehem* is good for learned stresses. For example, if you yelled at your cat for licking her coat when she was in her bed, she may not settle down when you are ready to go to bed yourself.
- *Mimulus* is for minimizing fears of all types: fear of the bath, fear of having ears or eyes cleaned, fear of wind, storms, etc.
- *Rock Rose* is used for present terror.
- *Vine* is for the overbearing pet.
- *Impatiens* quiets the pet that is always impatient and always a little nervous, despite your reassurance.

- *Aconite* addresses behavior that is the result of situations that produce sudden shock or fear.
- *Ignatia* helps to reduce symptoms related to grief or loss.

Unfortunately, nervousness, fear, or any intense emotion can reduce immune function and leave a pet very susceptible to toxins. Herbs such as *Valerian Root*, *Hops Flowers*, *Skullcap*, *Chamomile*, or *St. John's Wort* (which also helps balance hormones) help relax the pet, allowing them to rest more comfortably and sleep more deeply. (See Aggression.)

**Cancer** can often be the end result of unhealthy living, as "poor skin and coat" conditions will often accompany the other distressing symptoms of cancer. Cancerous cells rob the body of energy and cause increased susceptibility to toxins. I have seen many immune system problems, including Feline Leukemia, FIP, Tick Fever, Valley Fever and chronic anemia (possibly a pre-cancerous state), in pets originally diagnosed and treated chemically for "allergies" or chronic skin, ear, and eye problems. The constant stress on the body due to the symptoms themselves, as well as the chemicals and drugs used to treat them, weakens the animal's constitution and their recuperative abilities and encourages damaged cells to become cancerous.

Many of the symptom relief recommendations in this book are applicable to the treatment of cancerous conditions. In both cases, the underlying imbalance is likely to be in the immune system and skin conditions, allergies, or cancer are the symptoms. (See Immune Dysfunction.)

**Chewing** can drive both the pet and the owner nuts and is potentially very harmful to your pet. The constant stress of chewing and licking quickly leads to emotional and physical exhaustion, which further weakens the immune system. Treat chewing as a nervous habit rather than a symptom. First, you need to rule out any rashes, abrasions, cuts, flea or tick bites, etc. that may be triggering the chewing and address them topically. (See Allergy Reactions.)

Then utilize herbal and/or homeopathic remedies for irritability and nervousness. You will be amazed how effective these are, even if you do not believe that your pet has any emotional issues. Flower essences work well also.

### *Herbal Remedies for Chewing*

- *St. John's Wort* helps balance hormones and brain chemistry to provide a sense of well-being and calmness. It also acts as a sedative and improves pain relief.
- *Skullcap* supports the nervous system and helps control seizures and pain.
- *Chamomile* is an effective calmer and works well especially for digestive allergies possibly triggered by anxiety.
- *Wild Oats* is an excellent nerve tonic and helps rebalance the nervous system.
- *Valerian Root* is a calming and restorative herb.

### *Homeopathic Remedies for Chewing*

- *Aconite* addresses chewing that result from situations associated with sudden shock or fear and increased anxiety.
- *Ignatia* helps to reduce chewing related to grief or loss.
- *Arsenicum* can reverse an irritable disposition.

### *Flower Essences for Chewing*

- *Rock Rose*, *Chicory*, and *Holly* is beneficial for chewing.

**Constipation** is often associated with poor skin and coat conditions. Whereas diarrhea is often associated with toxic reactions, alternating constipation and diarrhea or constipation alone can also occur because of stress. Constipation can weaken the body because waste products have not been properly eliminated and toxins are reabsorbed from the colon into the bloodstream. Several factors can contribute to constipation, including medications like antibiotics and antihistamines often used for general skin conditions or allergies. First eliminate any possible culprits:

- hard to digest pet food ingredients, such as "plant cellulose" (often soy castings, peanut shells, or husks of any kind that are used as filler/fiber in pet food)
- lack of exercise, when an animal has been confined for six hours or more
- inadequate fluid intake
- excessive ingestion of fur or hair, due to licking and chewing
- ingestion of non-digestible objects such as rocks, rubber, bone, or feathers
- poor sources of dietary fiber

*Psyllium seed or husk*s are commonly used to regulate bowel movement, but, when used alone, often can be too harsh on the digestive tract. Combine it with other fruits and vegetables such as *carrots, apple fiber and pectin, guar gum* (a misunderstood, but excellent, source of natural fiber that swells to retain water), and *bran. Chinese mushrooms*, such as *Shiitake* and *Reishi,* which are also high in fiber, can help to reverse chronic colon conditions, including pre-cancerous growths. Cooked *oatmeal* added to meals or given alone with vegetable, fish, or meat broth, not only is high in fiber, but also has detoxifying properties to help eliminate old fecal material from the bowels. (See Digestive Disorders.)

**Cushing's Disease** is a serious malfunction of the adrenal gland, requiring a veterinarian's assistance. Many veterinarians have reported that when holistically addressing adrenal malfunction associated with skin and coat conditions, symptoms of Cushing's Disease have also improved.

Symptoms can include fatigue, hair color loss or poor coat growth, excessive shedding, slow tissue repair, and a droopy belly. The skin may be gray and leathery, resembling an elephant's skin. Within six months of natural support, this skin condition, which is generally believed to be irreversible, may be reduced in severity by up to eighty percent. (See Adrenal Malfunction.)

**Demodectic Mange** (See Skin Parasites.)

**Dermatitis.** Pets with nutritional deficiencies, allergies, or toxic reaction often have skin problems. Fleabites are also a common source of dermatitis. When the skin becomes irritated, inflamed, and itchy, pets begin to scratch, rub, chew, and lick themselves. The skin becomes so irritated and inflamed that other problems arise: hair loss, dandruff, greasy skin, pimples, and hot spots.

A *hot spot* is an irritated, open area of skin caused by scratching or biting, which can result in infection. Keep the area dry and clean. Clip away the hair around the hot spot to make it easier to clean and treat topically. If a pet has chronic dermatitis and has been exposed to many cycles of antibiotics, a staphylococcal infection may arise that is difficult to treat.

Avoid the use of coal tar-based or chemically medicated shampoos. Do not bathe too often when the skin is severely irritated, no more than every two to four weeks. Frequent whole body bathing can worsen the condition by drying out the skin, thereby encouraging greasy skin. (Body oils will try to replenish themselves quickly and heavily to counter such drying.) Instead, spot clean and disinfect the skin whenever needed.

Feed potent doses of a high-quality *garlic* supplement (500 mg. to 1000 mg. per day for small dogs and cats, up to 2000 mg. for medium- to large-sized dogs). In addition, Vitamin C and other nutritional support for allergies will do more to permanently clear up hot spots than topical treatment alone. (See Infections, Skin and Coat Problems.)

**Diarrhea** is often associated with toxic reactions, although it can manifest in pets suffering from other stresses, especially constant scratching and biting—all that nervous energy just churns up the bowel. *Psyllium seed or husk* is the most commonly used fiber to help regulate bowel movement, but often can be too harsh on the digestive tract, when used alone. Combine it with other fruit and vegetable fiber sources such as *carrots, apple fiber and pectin, guar gum*, and *bran.*

*Chinese mushrooms*, such as *Shiitake* and *Reishi* are high in fiber and are excellent for reversing chronic colon conditions, including pre-cancerous growths (which may be irritated and triggering the diarrhea).

Cooked *oatmeal*, added to meals or vegetable, fish, or meat broth, is an excellent source of fiber and has detoxifying properties to eliminate old fecal material from the bowels. Old fecal material can become toxic (especially with bacterial infection) and trigger the body's attempt to eliminate the irritation, resulting in the diarrhea.

Add to the oatmeal a high-quality *garlic* supplement (500 mg. to 1000 mg. per day for small dogs and cats, and up to 2000 mg. for medium- to large-sized dogs). This regimen will give your pet natural antibiotic support.

These homeopathic remedies are effective in relieving diarrhea and associated symptoms. Use *Arsenicum* for general symptoms, *China* for debilitating fluid loss, and *Nux Vomica* for vomiting and/or appetite loss.

Herbally, use *Yucca* and/or *Calendula Extract*, *Liquid Chlorophyll*, and *Slippery Elm Extract* or *Powder* to soothe irritated intestinal tissues. Be sure that fluid intake is maintained, as diarrhea can quickly dehydrate your pet. Add one-half teaspoon of *raw honey* per twenty pounds of body weight per day to fluids or herbal preparations. Honey is not only soothing to an irritated colon, it is antiseptic, and it provides energy for a weakened pet. (See Digestive Disorders.)

**Digestive Disorders** are very common in pets that exhibit skin and coat problems. They are associated with food and other environmental toxins. Aside from skin problems, lack of appetite, vomiting, stool changes, and hair balls are the most common complaints I hear from pet owners. The use of digestive enzymes can be beneficial in the short term, but you will have to address the actual imbalance for long-term symptom reversal.

Homeopathy is very effective in reversing acute stomachaches, liver inflammation, stool changes, and the underlying stress that often accompanies these digestive disorders.

### *Homeopathic Remedies for Digestive Disorders*

- *Arsenicum* is used for general digestive imbalances or toxicity and will alleviate most allergy-related digestive disorders, especially if there is liver or spleen involvement, or if the disorder has been triggered by a season of one dose per month of flea and tick control products.
- *Nux Vomica* also addresses the majority of digestive imbalances, including gas, vomiting, lack of appetite, or stool problems (especially alternating between constipation and diarrhea). It complements *Arsenicum*.
- *Carbo Veg* is helpful when the pet is overweight, has chronic stool problems, seems to have trouble digesting well, and

burps soon after eating. Is extremely beneficial when used with *Nux Vomica*, and is a good senior pet tonic.

- *Belladonna* is used for the sudden onset of gastrointestinal symptoms. After initial use, it should be tapered off slowly and then followed by a more specific remedy. It is also indicated for acute colic and pancreatic imbalances resulting in a "fatty" stool.
- *Urtica Urens* addresses a lack of appetite often accompanied by extensive itchy eruptions, hives, or serious welts. These afflictions, which are not responsive to *Apis* or *Sulphur*, often appear in conjunction with digestive or eliminatory problems, as well as dry skin aggravated by warmth or bathing. Digestive problems may also be associated with profuse discharges from mucous membranes, ears, and eyes. Symptoms may be localized to the right side of the body.
- *Phosphorus* is indicated if the digestive problems include great debilitation, fluid loss, frequent vomiting, or diarrhea soon after meals. Phosphorus quickly eliminates blood (from old fecal material, viral, or bacterial detoxification) or fatty mucus (from pancreatic imbalance) in the stool.
- *Podophyllum* can be used when profuse, offensive-smelling stools occur. Stool color may be yellowish or greenish. The stool is often completely liquid or begins formed and turns loose as the bowel movement progresses. The bowel movement can also be accompanied by dry heaves or gagging.
- *Pulsatilla* aids diarrhea or mucous-covered stools, which are often greenish in color. This stool will frequently change in character or color, even during the bowel movement. Diarrhea is likely to be worse at night or aggravated by warmth. Symptoms, such as nausea, vomiting, or diarrhea, are not too severe. Food is often the culprit, especially if it is high in animal fats or rancid ingredients. The offending food might be vomited up partially digested. The tongue may become coated with a thick white or yellowish material.
- *Ipecac* can quickly subdue vomiting, especially when it is related to food or ingested chemical allergies.
- *Colocynthis* is indicated for pets who are cramping or whose stomachs are rumbling. They want to lie on a hard surface or they will respond positively when you rub their belly. Movement, drinking, or eating will aggravate symptoms.

- *Bryonia* is indicated for pets that are cramping or whose stomachs rumble, but they avoid hard surfaces or respond in pain when their stomachs are rubbed. They may also exhibit arthritic pains as a result of an allergic reaction.
- *Mercurius* benefits pets who have marked upper digestive tract and liver involvement, especially when they feel pain when they are touched or lying on the right side. Stools may be whitish-gray or yellowish green. Often, pets are very irritable with swollen gums that bleed easily, and their tongues may be slightly swollen and coated with a yeast-like substance.
- *Lycopodium* is another excellent liver remedy, especially with back pain, gas, bloating, discomfort, and rumbling of the stomach soon after meals. These pets seem to fill up quickly after only a few bites of solid food.
- *China* supports pets that have chronic liver involvement with digestive imbalances who are very sensitive to touch and open air. They chill easily and seek to hide, especially after meals. Although they may crave cold water, it will cause them to burp up partially digested food.

Herbal remedies can support reversal of many symptoms associated with digestive disorders, can increase digestion or assimilation, and can stabilize appetite. Many pets cannot tolerate herbs on an empty stomach. In fact, the herbs may create some of the digestive distress. When pets have digestive upsets, it is best to give herbs with a little food until the herbs are better tolerated, or you might try to obtain better-quality herbs.

### *Herbal Remedies for Digestive Disorders*

- *Yucca Extract* provides natural steroidal saponins, which are effective in reducing inflammation in the digestive system, including the stomach and intestinal lining as well as the liver, gall bladder, spleen, and pancreas. A reduction in excessive peristalsis (the rhythmic undulation of the intestines that causes the movement of digested material through the colon) can help relieve diarrhea due to allergic and inflammatory responses. Intestinal pockets, ulcerations, and inflamed intestinal valves that block passages (often associated with allergy-related colitis) have also responded well to *Yucca* supplementation.

- *Garlic* is excellent for digestive complaints. Not only is it antiseptic and a natural antibiotic, it effectively supports proper digestion and colon health through its anti-parasitic and anti-yeast properties. Higher allicin contents are beneficial in reversing general diarrhea, flatulence, and fatty stool deposits.
- *Peppermint Leaf* or *Fenugreek Seed* helps to reduce intestinal gas, cramping, and colic, prevents fatty deposits, repairs digestive tissue ulcerations, and fights infection.
- *Dandelion Leaf* is an excellent tonic for the liver and gall bladder.
- *Siberian Ginseng Root* stimulates resistance against food or reactive allergies.
- *Milk Thistle Seed* supports proper liver function and detoxification.
- *Calendula Extract* contains therapeutic components that soothe sensitive and irritated digestive tissues, including the stomach and intestinal lining, as well as the liver, gall bladder, spleen, and pancreas.
- *Devil's Club Root Bark*, *Indian Jambul Seed*, *Dandelion Leaf and Root*, *Uva Ursi Leaf*, and *Turmeric Root* reduce the occurrence of soft, fatty, off-colored stools.
- *Cascara Sagrada Bark*, *Barberry Root*, *Senna Leaves*, *Rhubarb Root*, and *Cayenne* clean out the intestinal tract. A detoxified colon is fundamental to re-balancing the digestive system and increasing assimilation of nutrients necessary for proper skin and coat health. These herbs can also prevent or reverse parasitic infestation.
- *Fennel Seed*, *Ginger Root*, and *Anise Seed* relieve gas, cramping, and mucus while stimulating proper digestion and peristalsis.
- *Shiitake* and *Reishi Mushrooms* have been used by the Chinese for centuries to prevent and treat cancers associated with the digestive system. Colon cancer in particular responds well to their incredible healing properties. A dramatic reduction in

food sensitivities is often the result of long-term supplementation. (See Appetite Problems, Constipation, Diarrhea.)

**Ear Mites** (See Skin Parasites.)

**Ear problems** are common in many pets. The liver, a primary organ affected by allergens or toxins, has a relationship to the ears and eyes. As the liver becomes burdened, the ears begin to exhibit symptoms associated with allergy problems, becoming more prone to irritation from grasses, pollen, and molds, as well as foods and chemicals.

Symptoms often occur during warmer weather when dogs bathe and swim more. Water may become trapped in the ear channel, encouraging bacteria and yeast to grow there, leading to an ear infection. Foxtails and other foreign bodies may also become lodged in the ear. Always see if you can find anything in the ear and remove it prior to treatment. If needed, seek proper removal by a veterinarian.

Ears can be effectively cleaned with a homemade solution of *two ounces of distilled or purified water, one teaspoon of Witch Hazel, one teaspoon of White Vinegar and six drops of Calendula Extract.* Add an additional six drops of *Golden Seal Extract* if infection is suspected. Use a cotton ball to squeeze a little of this solution into the ear. Rub the outer base of the ear to massage the solution into any debris that needs to be removed (you may hear a slight suction-like noise inside the ear). Allow your pet to shake out their ears, then wipe out the rest of debris and fluid with a soft tissue wrapped around your finger. To avoid damage, do not insert anything down into the inner ear, but rather let the tissue absorb any impurities. Follow cleanings with an application of *Calendula Extract, Aloe Gel,* or *Vitamin E.* Use *Hypericum, Calendula,* or *Arnica Cream* around the flap and opening if pain is present.

Be careful not to use heavy, oil-based ingredients or vegetable oils, unless you are attempting to dissolve a foreign body or kill ear mites (see Skin Parasites). Although such oils may seem to be conditioning the ear and reducing irritation, they may also nurture a bacterial or yeast infection by providing a warm, moist, oxygen-free environment. For dogs with earflaps in the down position, tie them up over the head with an elastic hair band to encourage air circulation. Tying the ears up for as little as one hour a day can reduce bacterial or yeast growth and encourage healing.

To dissolve a suspected foreign body which is not creating severe pain or bleeding, *warm up two tablespoons of garlic-flavored cooking oil* (which will help discourage bacterial growth) or use soybean oil and add a capsule of *garlic extract* to it. Add six drops each of *Golden Seal* and *Mullein Extract* and 200 IUs of *Vitamin E* to the garlic oil. Drip the mixture down into the ear with an eyedropper, spoon, or cotton ball. Keep it in the ear for as long as your pet will tolerate it, and massage the base of the ear to loosen the object further before flushing the ear out with the cleaning solution. Repeat several times per day until the object is removed, usually within a day or two. This will dissolve hardened debris as well as many plant particles. Never force fluid into the ear, or you may drive the object further in, making it harder for you to remove safely.

*Grapefruit Extract eardrops* can be applied after cleaning the ear to fight bacterial and yeast infections. *Mullein and Garlic oil eardrops* are also excellent for irritated and infected ears.

Avoid alcohol-based products, which can irritate the ears further—unless you suspect water is trapped in the ear canal, in which case a few drops of pure alcohol can dry up the fluid residue. Don't worry about the alcohol found in herbal extracts—very little alcohol remains by the final dilution. Avoid glycerin-based herbal extracts in general, unless your pet has sensitivity to alcohol. I have found them to be less therapeutically potent than alcohol-based products.

Proper grooming is also beneficial for keeping the ears free of infection or waxy build-up. Many breeds, such as Poodles, Terriers, and Cocker Spaniels, grow hair in close proximity to the ear opening, and sometimes even in it. You must pull the hair from in the ear and clip the outer areas short, to help air circulate. Many dog breeds that are prone to ear infections have a closed flap ear, rather than a standing flap ear. A standing ear allows air to circulate, drying ears quickly and thoroughly, thus avoiding infection.

### *Herbal Remedies for Ear Problems*

- *Garlic* is vital to eliminating ear problems. Use a high-potency supplement for basic antibacterial support. Because it is high in natural sulfur, garlic helps heal irritated tissue and reverse eruptions and irritations.
- *Yucca Extract* works as well as steroids to reduce inflammatory responses. (See Allergic Reactions.)
- *Spilanthes Flowering Tops and Roots*, *Oregon Grape Root*, and *Myrrh Gum* work well together for more serious yeast and/or fungal infections.
- *Red Clover Blossoms*, *Stinging Nettle Leaf*, and *Cleavers* help soothe irritated tissue, often seen in severely itchy ears with rashes or tiny pimples inside and around the ear.
- *Turmeric Root*, *Black Catechu*, *Grindelia Floral Buds*, and *Lobelia* is a combination that protects the liver from circulating antigens and allergens, thereby reducing ear infections and irritations associated with airborne and food-related allergies. Ear problems, particularly those accompanied by digestive disorders, respond well to this combination.
- *Eyebright*, *Bayberry Root*, *Calamus Root*, *Golden Seal Root*, and *Stinging Nettle Leaf* is excellent for ear infections directly related to grass or pollen sensitivities, which are often accompanied by eye irritation or discharge. Symptoms include very itchy, blotchy, infected ear tissue, often visibly swollen.

- *Echinacea*, *Red Root*, *Baptisia Root*, *Thuja Leaf*, and *Prickly Ash Bark* clean the blood and lymphatic systems, and activate the body's immune response. This combination is beneficial when the ear condition is associated with auto immune dysfunction, which is chronic and difficult to address. Other symptoms that respond well to this combination includes ear flap hematoma or blood blisters, which are often the result of trauma due to scratching.
- *Sheep Sorrel*, *Burdock Root*, *Slippery Elm*, and *Turkey Rhubarb Root* combined are often the key to chronic symptom reversal. (See Immune System Dysfunction.)

Nutritional and herbal supplementation works to reverse systemic weaknesses and reduces symptom reoccurrence. Homeopathic remedies can quickly reverse acute symptoms associated with ear-related allergies.

### *Homeopathic Remedies for Ear Problems*

- *Arsenicum and Apis* combined are effective for sensitivities to airborne allergens, especially itchy ears.
- *Silica* and *Arnica* combined are effective when a hematoma (large blood blister) has formed on the ear flap. The *Silica* expels the blister, while the *Arnica* helps heal it without pain. (See Abscesses.)
- *Graphites* works well to alleviate foul-smelling discharge.
- *Hepar Sulph* helps inflamed ears with discharge.
- *Mercurius* relieves boils and hematoma found on the external ear canal, and is good for reversing thick, yellow discharge that is often foul-smelling and bloody.
- *Rhus Tox* is indicated for chronic ear infections. It works well with *Arsenicum*.
- *Hypericum* can be used if ears are extremely sensitive to touch.
- *Aconite* supports the pet that has become overly sensitive about being petted on the head during or after being treated for ear infections.

If the ear seems more irritated, begins to bleed profusely, becomes unbearably painful, or develops a severe discharge, and is non-responsive to home treatment within a few days, then seek out veterinarian care immediately. Do not take ear problems lightly, as chronic inflammation and infections can lead to permanent damage, resulting in deafness. Reliance on a chemically based, medicated ear wash or drops can also permanently damage the sensitive tissues of the ear. (See Infections, Skin and Coat Problems, and Skin Parasites.)

**Eczema** (See Skin and Coat Problems.)

**Emotional Problems** (See Behavioral Problems.)

**Eye Problems** are almost always involved in toxic responses and often accompany ear symptoms, as both the eyes and ears are indicative of liver function. Allergens and toxins can overwhelm the liver. Resistance to airborne sensitivities, in particular, is compromised. Check your pet's eyes daily, and wipe away any matter present. Always address eye problems quickly, as chronic irritation or infection can permanently damage the eye, possibly leading to cataract formation and even blindness.

To clean away discharge, use a warm, damp cotton cloth. Always use distilled water on the cloth. Wipe in the direction of the eyelashes to avoid further irritating the eye. Start in the inside corner; allow your pet to close the eye before gently wiping lightly downwards towards the outside corner.

To remove heavy matter or copious discharge in and around the eye, use a warm, wet cotton pad or ultra-soft cotton paper towel. Hold it gently against the eye, allowing it time to soften any hardened matter. Gently wipe the inside of the lid to remove discharge on the eyeball, being careful not to introduce any dirt or crust into the eye. Then remove the remaining matter on the outside lashes. Repeat as often as needed. Do not allow the eye to remain crusted-over and shut. This will encourage infection and can damage the eye or tear duct permanently.

Follow cleaning with an application of natural eye drops made by diluting six drops of *Calendula Extract* in a couple of ounces of distilled water. For very irritated or dry eyes, apply a few drops of natural *Vitamin E oil*, every other day, directly to the inside of the lower eyelid. Be careful not to scratch the eye. Blinking will disperse the Vitamin E. A few drops of *Golden Seal Extract* can also be added to eye drops, if infection is present. This will also help to open up tear ducts, and encourage natural lubrication. (See Infections.)

### *Herbal Remedies for Eye Problems*

Always supplement with herbs to strengthen and cleanse the eye, increase resistance to allergens and infections, and support anti-inflammatory and antihistamine action. Proper nutritional and herbal supplementation can prevent and even reverse cataracts, a common side effect of chronic eye irritation.

- *Yucca Extract* works as well as steroids in reducing inflammatory responses. (See Allergic Reactions.)
- *Chinese Ephedra*, *Mullein Leaves*, and *Lobelia* is a natural antihistamine combination, which quickly reduces acute responses that result in itchy eyes and tearing. It is excellent for short-term symptom suppression and gives other herbs and nutrients a chance to build up the body.
- *Eyebright*, *Bayberry Root*, *Calamus Root*, *Golden Seal Root*, and *Stinging Nettle Leaf* address very itchy, dry eyes that are often visibly swollen or weepy due to infection.
- *Red Clover Blossoms*, *Stinging Nettle Leaf*, and *Cleavers* soothe irritated tissue, which can manifest as severely inflamed, itchy

eyes with rashes or tiny pimples around the eyes, face, and ears. It can help prevent and eliminate tiny eyelid cysts and is excellent for mange-reactive eye sensitivities.

- *Echinacea*, *Red Root*, *Baptisia Root*, *Thuja Leaf*, and *Blue Flag Root* clean the blood and lymphatic systems and activate the body's immune response. This combination is beneficial with difficult to address eye conditions that may be associated with autoimmune dysfunction. Other symptoms that respond well to this combination include tiny blood blisters or cysts around the lids that are often the result of trauma due to scratching.
- *Sheep Sorrel*, *Burdock Root*, *Slippery Elm*, and *Turkey Rhubarb Root* can be the key to chronic symptom reversal. (See Immune System Dysfunction.)

### *Homeopathic Remedies for Eye Problems*

- *Arsenicum and Apis* are a good combination for sensitivities to airborne allergens, especially itchy, runny eyes.
- *Silica and Hypericum* work together to help unblock tear ducts. Also follow directions for abscesses if needed.
- *Euphrasia* encourages tearing to reduce dryness and irritability.
- *Aconite* is beneficial when the eyes are severely inflamed and red with hard, swollen lids. Eye conditions that seem aggravated by wind and sunlight and tend to tear profusely respond to *Aconite*.
- *Pulsatilla* is indicated for creamy, profuse eye discharges.
- *Hypericum and Arnica* should be used if there is injury and pain due to scratching or chronic rubbing of the eyes.

**Fatty Tumors** (See Skin and Coat Problems.)

**Fleas** (See Skin Parasites.)

**Fleabite Dermatitis** (See Skin and Coat Problems.)

**Hair Loss** (See Skin and Coat Problems.)

**Heart Problems**, such as a rapid heartbeat, can accompany chronic chemical reactions, which stress the heart due to powerful surges of histamine and adrenaline. Excessive panting can mistakenly be attributed to allergies, yet possibly indicate a more serious heart condition, so be sure to report any changes in breathing patterns or weakness with exercise to your veterinarian.

### *Homeopathic Remedies for Heart Problems*

If heart problems are primarily affected by chemical reactions, then homeopathic remedies should quickly address them.

- *Aconite* is beneficial when labored breathing and tumultuous heart action follow allergic response, or when heart inflammation is suspected.
- *Arsenicum* is indicated when weakness is triggered by a chemical reaction, particularly by vaccination, topical skin treatment, or pest control products. The heart may fluctuate between rapid and labored beating.
- *Iberis* helps regulate an irregular heartbeat and reduce palpitations.

**Hot Spots** (See Skin and Coat Problems.)

**Immune System Dysfunction** is often the root of poor skin and coat conditions. It is vital that you address and support proper immune function. Unfortunately, it is common to see pets develop more serious disease, such as cancer, after struggling for years with poor condition and symptoms. Many people have also reported an increase or sudden development of skin irritations after the pet has been treated medically for another condition, such as kidney problems. In each case, the underlying weakness is the immune system, and the best way to reverse most symptoms is to strengthen the immune system first.

*Vitamin C, A, B-Complex*, and *E* cannot be surpassed for their immune-enhancing capabilities. Several other vitamins, minerals (such as *Zinc*, *Selenium*, and *Chromium)*, and amino acids can enhance the efficacy of these nutrients, so a properly balanced and therapeutically potent multiple supplement is essential.

In addition, several herbal and homeopathic remedies support resistance to antigens or infections, reduce catabolic waste (responsible for many skin and digestive symptoms), and eliminate damaged or mutated cells, which are often responsible for a weakened immune response, and the genesis of cancerous cells.

### *Herbal Remedies for Immune Dysfunction*

Herbal extracts, preferably organic and standardized (which have a stronger, guaranteed potency) should be diluted in purified water, tuna water, or apple juice and given on an empty stomach for optimum therapeutic response. If your pet is suffering from digestive disorders, herbs may be better tolerated when given with meals.

- *Sheep Sorrel*, *Burdock Root*, *Slippery Elm*, and *Turkey Rhubarb Root* is an indigenous herbal remedy to eliminate catabolic waste and stimulate the immune system. Chronic cases often need this foundation for detoxification and increased resistance. Several dog breeds, such as Dalmatians, Cockers, and German Shepherds, and Siamese or Persian cats, who suffer from genetically induced chronic immune weaknesses, often fail to recover until this combination is introduced. This combination is a good preventative herbal remedy.
- *Echinacea* and *Golden Seal Root* are nature's antibiotics. They promote resistance to viral, bacterial, yeast, and fungal infection while stimulating the immune system in general. These natural antibiotics cleanse the blood, lymphatic system, liver, and kidneys. They can be used topically for the reversal of

abscesses, gangrene, and pus discharge, and also to open up blocked tear ducts.

- *Astragalus Root* helps tone and stimulate the spleen, an important immune system organ. It fights infection, helps restore appetite, and reduces fatigue and diarrhea resulting from infection. It is also useful for prolapsed conditions of the anus and impacted anal glands. It acts as a diuretic to flush wastes, reduce edema, and discharge pus, and it increases metabolism and aids the adrenals.
- *Pau d'Arco* is beneficial for the whole body. It stimulates the immune system, heals wounds, combats infections, kills viruses, and is effective against cancers (including lupus and leukemia), cysts, and tumors. Use it internally and topically for ringworm, hot spots, eczema, psoriasis, and staphylococcal infections. It provides general support and can reverse cystitis, colitis, gastritis, diabetes, liver, and kidney weaknesses. *Pau d'Arco* relieves arthritic pain and is easier for sick, weakened, or older pets to tolerate than *Golden Seal Root*.
- *Lomatium Root*, *Echinacea Root*, *Spilanthes*, *Chinese Schizandra Berry*, and *Licorice Root* promote strong anti-viral activity and have immune-enhancing properties. This combination of herbs enhances cellular immunity and liver function to protect healthy cells from antigens and viral infection. They are indicated in cases of chronic viral infections that have not responded well to medications, or where the liver may be inflamed. This combination can be used with *Astragalus* for debilitating or chronic infection.
- *Echinacea*, *Red Root*, *Baptisia Root*, *Thuja Leaf*, and *Prickly Ash Bark* drain toxins and infection from the blood and lymphatic system, while activating the body's immune response. Symptoms that respond well to this combination include: autoimmune conditions and catabolic waste build-up, tiny blood blisters, pimples/feline acne, skin ulcerations, lymphatic engorgement, chronic infection, tumor growth, cysts, fluid cysts, cancer, reactive arthritis, and wasting disease.
- *Spilanthes Leaf and Root*, *Grape Root*, *Juniper Berry*, *Usnea Lichen*, and *Myrrh Gum* combined is a powerful anti-fungal and anti-yeast agent. This combination is beneficial in reducing Valley Fever spore infestation. It helps the immune

system respond to yeast overgrowth, vaginal infection, penis discharge, and ringworm.

### *Homeopathic Remedies for Immune Dysfunction*

Homeopathic remedies can facilitate the immune system's response to a specific toxin, allergen, bacterial, viral, yeast infection, or parasitic infestation, although they should never be relied upon solely to address immune imbalance. If an animal is severely debilitated, you may have to use a homeopathic remedy along with nutritional and herbal supplementation.

- *Arsenicum* promotes detoxification and elimination through the liver and kidneys and stimulates other organs and glands responsible for proper immune response. *Arsenicum* prepares the body to utilize immune-enhancing nutrients.
- *Gelsemium* should be used at the first signs of disease, especially fever. Use this remedy for pets that seem very needy and want to be held when they begin to feel ill, or have had a relapse after a long, debilitating illness and slow recovery.
- *Echinacea* is good for reoccurring boils, intolerance of insect bites, and lymphatic engorgement. It helps address the fatigue often associated with immune problems.
- *Sweet Chestnut* is a flower remedy that addresses deep despair and anguish often experienced by a pet after a long illness.

**Infections** can be addressed through herbal extracts, preferably organic and standardized (stronger, guaranteed potency). Extracts should be diluted in purified water or apple juice and given on an empty stomach for optimum therapeutic response. If your pet is suffering from digestive disorders, herbs may be better tolerated when given with meals. If this is the case, then increase the dose slightly to help assimilation.

### *Herbal Remedies for Infections*

- *Sheep Sorrel, Burdock Root, Slippery Elm*, and *Turkey Rhubarb Root* is an indigenous herbal remedy for pets suffering from chronic or severe infections. Genetically or medically compromised animals need this foundation for detoxification of catabolic waste and increased resistance to re-infection. (See Immune Dysfunction.)

- *Echinacea* and *Golden Seal Root* (See Immune Dysfunction.)
- *Astragalus Root* aids the adrenals, to support the body while the body combats infections. (See Immune Dysfunction.)
- *Pau d'Arco* kills viruses and helps reduce fever. It provides excellent general support and can reverse weakness from chronic infection and long-term medication. (See Immune Dysfunction.)
- *Lomatium Root*, *Echinacea Root*, *Spilanthes*, *Chinese Schizandra Berry*, and *Licorice Root* enhance anti-viral activity. (See Immune Dysfunction.)
- *Echinacea*, *Red Root*, *Baptisia Root*, *Thuja Leaf*, and *Prickly Ash Bark* drain the blood and lymphatic systems, while activating the body's immune response to fight infection. (See Immune Dysfunction.)
- *Spilanthes Leaf and Root*, *Grape Root*, *Juniper Berry*, *Usnea Lichen*, and *Myrrh Gum* combined, are very powerful anti-fungal and anti-yeast agents. (See Immune Dysfunction.)

Homeopathic remedies are not, in my opinion, very effective in fighting infection by themselves, and should be used to address acute secondary symptoms. (See Abscesses, Immune System Dysfunction, Skin and Coat Problems.)

**Lick Granuloma** can develop on the body, especially around the lower legs and feet, after chronic trauma through licking has occurred. A hard knot slowly develops that is often the primary spot for a pet's focus. Therefore, it is commonly thought to be simply obsessive behavior, and the condition is not addressed until the granuloma appears. Once the licking has become chronic, it has also become obsessive behavior and is not addressed during treatment. Although the "trigger" itself has been suppressed, compulsive licking of the area will help continue the symptom cycle by re-irritating the skin. Although surgical removal of the granuloma is often the suggested course of veterinary treatment, I discourage it because the granuloma can return with a vengeance and is then more likely to become cancerous.

**Licking** is a serious concern for many pet owners. Excessive licking is not only irritating to the owner; it will quickly exhaust the pet. The pet's vital healing energy is redirected to address this fatigue, instead of supporting tissue repair and immune stimulation.

Although normal daily self-grooming includes licking the body clean, obsessive and chronic licking can lead to hairballs (see Digestive Disorders), skin eruptions (see Skin and Coat Problems), and growths (see Lick Granuloma). Homeopathic *Arsenicum* works the best for constant licking, especially when a build-up of urea is involved. *St. John's Wort* and *Chamomile* help reduce the anxiety often associated with excessive licking. Try Flower Essences, such as *Rescue* or *Mimulus*, which are good for obsessive behavior. (See Abscesses, Allergic Reactions, Chewing, and Digestive Disorders.)

**Liver Problems** are often at the root of skin and coat symptoms. The liver can become burdened and congested by yeast or chemical allergy-relief products. Immediately eliminate all yeast from your pet's diet, supplements, treats, or pest control products if you suspect liver disorder.

### *Herbal Remedies for Liver Problems*

- *Yucca* and *Garlic Extract* are excellent for promoting detoxification of the liver and help reduce general inflammation and organ congestion. (See Allergic Reactions.)

- *Milk Thistle Seed, Yellow Dock Root, Burdock Root, Echinacea Root, Sarsaparilla Root,* and *Oregon Grape Root* work together to promote a healthy liver. These herbs address improper fatty acid metabolism, detoxify the liver and blood, reduce bacterial and hormonal disorders associated with poor liver function, and alleviate chronic skin conditions.
- *Lomatium Root, Echinacea Root, Spilanthes, Chinese Schizandra Berry,* and *Licorice Root* target cellular immunity and liver function to protect healthy cells from antigens and viral infection. (See Immune System Dysfunction.)
- *Echinacea, Red Root, Baptisia Root, Thuja Leaf,* and *Prickly Ash Bark* act as blood and lymphatic cleansers, reducing liver toxicity. (See Immune System Dysfunction.)
- *Sheep Sorrel, Burdock Root, Slippery Elm,* and *Turkey Rhubarb Root* is good for catabolic waste elimination and liver stimulation. (See Immune System Dysfunction, Anemia, Digestive Disorders.)

**Mange** (See Skin Parasites.)

**Mites** (See Skin Parasites.)

**Pancreatitis** (See Digestive Disorders.)

**Pregnancy** is mentioned here because many pets first develop skin and coat symptoms while pregnant. This is understandable, given the amount of toxins produced by supporting the growing litter. Some pets quickly regain their former sheen, although it is more common to find pregnancy was the genesis of chronic skin and coat problems for many animals. Please do not breed any pets that have a history of immune-related conditions such as allergies, or you probably will pass on this genetic weakness. Research any herbal supplements you use during pregnancy, since many herbs can be dangerous for both mother and babies.

### *Herbs to Avoid during Pregnancy*

- *Angelica, Golden Seal, Pennyroyal* can cause uterine contractions.
- *Mugwort, Wormwood, Rue* also stimulate contractions.
- *Barberry, Cascara Sagrada* can be too strong a laxative during pregnancy.
- *Buchu, Juniper Berry* are strong diuretics and can be too dehydrating.
- *Ephedra (Ma Huang)* is too strong an antihistamine to use during pregnancy, although when it is used as a tea, it may help respiration without stress.

If you suspect that your pet is pregnant and exhibits symptoms, use the alternative fasting program and a well-balanced nutritional supplement with large amounts of Vitamins B and C.

Administer *safe* herbal remedies. Homeopathic remedies are safe to give during pregnancy. You must expect the unexpected during pregnancy. Be careful, always keep a close eye on the mother-to-be for any reactions or stress so you can alter her feeding and supplementation as needed before there is a crisis.

### *Beneficial and Safe Herbs to Use during Pregnancy*

- *Garlic* is supportive and nourishing to the growing babies.
- *Yucca Extract* is a safe alternative to steroid use. (See Allergic Reactions.)
- *Ginger Root* and *Peppermint* will control digestive upsets well.
- *Stinging Nettles* is a wonderful antihistamine, a good alternative to *Ephedra*.
- *Burdock Root* helps reverse anemia and strengthens the immune system.
- *Yellow Dock* improves iron assimilation and skin conditions.
- *Bilberry* promotes kidney function and detoxification.
- *Echinacea Leaf* is a safe immune stimulant and herbal antibiotic.

### *Beneficial and Safe Homeopathic Remedies to Use during Pregnancy*

- *Arsenicum*, *Apis*, and *Nux Vomica* are safe for detoxification, digestive upsets, excessive licking, scratching, and skin eruptions.
- *Nux Vomica* is good for old symptoms that have recurred with pregnancy.
- *Pulsatilla* relieves stress-related diarrhea during pregnancy, especially if pet is highly excitable or suffers exhaustion from symptoms that are worse during the day.
- *Alumina* is used for abnormal cravings, small hard knotty stool, or difficulty passing stool of any shape or consistency.
- *Sepia* is used for threatened abortion proceeded by severe allergies.
- *Phosphorus* helps reduce uterine bleeding.

**Ringworm** (See Skin Parasites.)

**Skin and Coat Problems** and related conditions often occur together. The skin, the largest eliminatory organ, can manifest many symptoms due to toxicity.

**Eczema, Hot Spots, Pimples, Cysts, Fatty Tumors,** and **Warts** can be reversed with a combination of herbs including *Red Clover, Stinging Nettle Leaf, Cleavers Herb, Yellow Dock Root, Burdock Root,* and *Yarrow Flowers.* Homeopathically, *Apis* addresses rashes and general irritation, which result in scratching or rubbing. *Thuja* and/or *Arsenicum* help eliminate warts, cysts, and fatty growths, as does *Calcarea Carb. Silica* works to eliminate growths under the skin, including cysts, abscesses, or ulcers. *Hepar Sulph* is indicated for weepy, painful areas.

**Greasy Coat** or **Offensive Odors** can be addressed through proper grooming and an antiseptic rinse. To make an antiseptic rinse, cut up one lemon (rind and all). Boil it in one pint of distilled water for five minutes. Then cover and simmer for twenty minutes. Let it sit in the water overnight. Strain in the morning and refrigerate. Add twenty drops of *Golden Seal Extract* or *Grapefruit Extract* if needed for infection control. Homeopathic *Psorinum* is beneficial when the skin has an acrid odor with discharging pustules or hot spots that are slow to heal. *Psorinum* reduces production of sebaceous glands, which is associated with a greasy coat and sebaceous cysts.

**Dry Coat, Dandruff, Cracked Skin,** and **Thin Skin** should be addressed with herbal formulas containing *Milk Thistle Seed* (for liver toxicity), *Yellow Dock Root* (improves fatty acid metabolism), *Burdock Root* (purifies blood), *Echinacea Root* (antibacterial, anti-ehrlichiosis), *Sarsaparilla Root* (for disorders associated with hormonal balance), and *Oregon Grape Root* (aids liver metabolism). *Arsenicum* is a good general homeopathic choice, while *Sepia* works well on irritations (especially cracked toes and feet) that itch badly with no relief from scratching. *Psorinum* can be used for a dirty and dingy coat that is brittle and lackluster. Topical application of *Jojoba oil* conditioner can also help reduce dryness temporarily, while herbs and nutrients build up in the body and reverse the underlying imbalance.

**Hair Loss, Poor Coat Condition,** and **Excessive Scratching** respond well to *Turmeric Root*, *Black Catechu*, *Grindelia Flowers*, *Licorice Root*, *Ginkgo Leaf*, *African Devil's Claw*, *Yarrow*, and *Lobelia*. Homeopathic *Arsenicum* is best suited for general hair loss. *Sulphur* addresses ringworm or other circular-patch irritations, often the cause of scratching and hair loss.

Proper grooming is of paramount importance for stimulating dead coat and skin removal and supporting circulation. Grooming will bring more nutrients to the skin and coat for tissue repair. A daily brushing, followed by a rubdown with a damp terry cloth towel can work wonders. (See Allergic Reactions.)

**Skin Parasites** can trigger your pet's poor skin and coat condition. It is prudent to have your pet examined to find out whether a skin parasite is present, so that it may be addressed if parasites are one of the underlying problems. Avoid the use of medicated or chemical-based topical pest control treatments, which can possibly depress the immune system and increase your pet's sensitivity to allergic reactions.

Whatever the cause of the skin and coat problems, immune system imbalance needs to be addressed. Healthy, non-toxic pets do not encourage infestation. Waste products exuded through the skin will invite and feed fleas and ticks. Yeast, commonly used to ward off fleas and ticks, may become toxic to the liver, increasing instances of infestation. Earwax and debris can also form, which provides an area for bacterial and yeast infections and attracts ear mites.

### *Common Parasitic Infestations Associated with Skin and Coat Conditions*

*Demodex Mites* are vicious skin parasites that borrow down into the epidermis, causing *Demodactic Mange*, which results in a great deal of discomfort and irritation. Scratching and chewing can quickly lead to infection with discharge. Puppies and chronically ill or elderly pets are particularly susceptible to *Demodactic Mange*, especially those animals who have recently been vaccinated.

Puppies are most often first infested by the bitch, who may not show signs of the mange but may be infested with mites. The pups become symptomatic after their immune systems are compromised. Although they may grow out of it, puppies can be very debilitated by chronic mange. Though it can be widespread on the body, it is often located on the head and neck where it causes skin inflammation and spreading patterns of rashes and hair loss.

Topically, treat daily with a solution of twelve drops *Grapefruit Extract*, six drops each of *Tea Tree Oil, Golden Seal Root Extract* and *Pau d'Arco Extract*, two drops of *Yucca Extract*, and three tablespoons of fresh squeezed lemon juice diluted in two ounces of *Witch Hazel* and four ounces of distilled water. Let mange area air dry and leave it uncovered.

*Sarcoptes* are a type of mite that causes *Sarcoptic Mange* in weakened or chronically ill pets. Referred to as "scabies," these mites can burrow into human flesh as well in order to lay eggs. It is vital that you treat the whole household if symptoms appear. Symptoms can include itchy rashes localized around the ears, elbows, and hocks. Scratching can be intense, so *Yucca Extract* should be given orally to reduce inflammation. (See Allergic Reactions.) For a topical solution, see the advice given for *Demodex Mites*.

*Ear Mites or Otodectes* are tiny, white spider-like pests. They are practically impossible to see with the naked eye. They leave a trail of digested blood and debris in the ear, which resembles finely ground pepper and results in a gritty discharge. To dissolve a suspected infestation that is not creating severe pain or bleeding, warm up two tablespoons of *garlic-flavored cooking oil*, to discourage bacterial growth—or use soybean oil and add a capsule of garlic extract—with six drops each of *Golden Seal* and *Mullein Extract*, and 200 IUs of *Vitamin E*. Apply with a dropper, spoon, or cotton ball, dripping it down into the ear. Allow it to set for as long as your pet will tolerate, at least one-half hour, if possible, to suffocate the mites. Finish by massaging the base of the ear to loosen the debris further before flushing the ear out with a cleaning solution. Repeat several times per day until all the mites are removed, usually within a day or two. (See Ears.)

*Fleas* and *Ticks* can not only create a lot of problems related to skin disorders, but also make treating the symptoms impossible if infestation is allowed to continue. They weaken and can infect your pet with more serious disease. *Diatomaceous earth* (tiny, ground-up fossils which dehydrate the pest's outer coating and therefore kill it) can be an effective barrier between your home or yard and the pests. Clean bedding and pet well with a natural insecticide shampoo and follow with a natural dip. Follow all directions carefully. Groom daily to help remove pests, dead skin and coat, and also to make skin treatments easier.

*Ringworm* is a fungal infection often mistaken for a parasite. It can create many of the same symptoms, such as skin inflammation, itching, and hot spots. Ringworm looks like a small, circular area with hair loss and irritation. Scratching can lead to bacterial infection. Treat it topically with mange solution or apply *lavender oil* to those areas.

Once you have correctly identified the problem and specifically addressed it, those symptoms that are associated with your pet's condition may begin to reverse themselves. Seek additional herbal or homeopathic support when needed.

*Red Clover Blossoms, Stinging Nettle Leaf, Cleavers Herb, Yellow Dock Root, Burdock Root, Yarrow Flowers, Plantain Leaf and Corm, Licorice Root*, and *Prickly Ash Bark* purify the blood and drain excess lymphatic fluids. They are indicated for skin disorders such as mange.

*Spilanthes Leaf and Root, Grape Root, Juniper Berry, Usnea Lichen, and Myrrh Gum* can be effectively used together to reverse ringworm, as can *Sarsaparilla*. These herbs can be used topically and internally. (See Ear Problems, Immune System Dysfunction, Infection, Skin and Coat Problems.)

**Stomach Problems** (See Digestive Disorders.)

**Ticks** (See Skin Parasites.)

**Thyroid Problems** can be very common in animals that exhibit poor skin and coat condition, especially with chronic infections. Often, the thyroid problem can be caused by previous cycles of steroid medications, the drugs most commonly used to suppress allergy-related symptoms.

Although I do prefer to rely on nutrients and glandulars to balance improperly functioning glands, I recommend that you read *Pet Allergies: Remedies for an Epidemic* by Alfred J. Plechner, DVM, and Martin Zucker if you are interested in studying allergies in greater depth. If you like the book, please lend your copy to your veterinarian.

Testing for hormonal or cortisol levels is beneficial. Utilize medication when appropriate for you and your animal, especially if nothing else seems to work.

*Raw glandulars with thyroid* and supportive ones such as adrenal and pituitary glands, plus proper nutrition, can often reverse thyroid weakness and rebalance function. *Yucca*, in the standardized extract form, seems to help the thyroid respond more quickly to nutritional support.

Herbal therapy with *Bladderwrack*, *Thuja leaf*, and *Blue Flag Root* is good for goiter and thyroid hypo-activity, while *Bugleweed*, *Motherwort*, *Lemon Balm*, and *Melissa* are appropriate for hyperactivity.

**Vaccinations** can trigger an allergic reaction and weaken the immune system enough to lower resistance to toxins in general. If you suspect that this is the case, then use homeopathic *Arsenicum* and *Thuja* in frequent daily doses until symptoms begin to reverse themselves. Symptoms can include lethargy, excessive shedding, digestive upsets including loss of appetite, and fever. You may also see a discharge from the anus, the nose, the eyes, or the injection site within twelve hours of the shots. Rashes, hot spots, and hair loss, in addition to loss of overall condition, may follow for years.

To use these remedies as a preventive and to lessen the likelihood of a reaction, begin dosing a few days prior to the shots. Avoid giving yearly vaccinations during the seasons your pet is most symptomatic, or avoid vaccinations altogether by researching homeopathic nosodes made from the actual diseases, such as parvo or FIP. I have had great success with this type of homeopathic protection.

**Valley Fever** is a serious, often fatal, fungal infestation, found in the arid southwestern states. Pets with chronic skin and coat problems are most prone to Valley Fever. The fungal spores grow deep in dry desert soil and are released by any type of digging. The spores are inhaled or absorbed through the skin. Treatment with chemical anti-fungal agents, such as *Nizoral*, often suppresses symptoms only to have them return with a vengeance once medication is ceased.

The side effects of anti-fungal drugs can be permanently damaging to the liver and kidneys, as well as causing suppression of the immune system. Therefore, it is not uncommon for pets being treated for Valley Fever to develop skin and coat symptoms. The best way to reverse these symptoms is to address the underlying cause.

Herbal treatment is effective in reversing the fungal count and stimulating the immune system, which can result in improved skin and coat condition. Often, the count may end up in the low end (for example, 1:4), but it will never reach zero since the body retains antibodies. Nevertheless, a holistically supported pet can remain free of symptoms or weakness, regardless of this "positive" titer count.

***Herbal Remedies for Valley Fever***

- *Garlic Extract* is anti-fungal. Use it for Valley Fever and related symptoms, lack of appetite, and other digestive disorders.
- *Yucca Extract* relieves the inflammatory response often associated with Valley fever, since the spore infestation can settle in the brain, lungs, bones, and joints as well as the skin.
- *Spilanthes Leaf and Root, Grape Root, Juniper Berry, Usnea Lichen*, and *Myrrh Gum*, combined, are very powerful anti-fungal and anti-yeast agents, and are beneficial in reducing Valley Fever spore infestation and secondary infections.

**Vomiting** (See Digestive Disorders.)

**Warts** (See Skin and Coat Problems.)

**Weight Problems** are not uncommon in pets also struggling with poor skin and coat conditions. Improper digestion and assimilation (also at the root of dis-ease) can interfere with the body's ability to utilize calories properly for energy. The brain is responsible for deciding if the body is being fed enough. If nutrients are not available to the blood through proper assimilation, the brain will think that the body is starving. It then decides to store calories as fat, rather than use them as energy to repair tissue and support the immune system. Pets who suffer great anxiety or debilitation along with their skin conditions can also have trouble maintaining proper weight, regardless of what they are fed.

Herbs, such as *Chickweed, Safflower Flowers, Burdock Root, Parsley, Licorice Root, Hawthorne Berries, Fennel*, and *Cayenne* work together to melt pounds away naturally and rebalance the digestive tract for greater assimilation.

*Siberian Ginseng, Chinese Schizandra Berry, Damiana Leaf, Kola Nut, Wild Oats, Skullcap*, and *Prickly Ash* work synergistically to restore integrity to the adrenal glands and promote weight gain and maintenance. This combination helps a pet adapt to and counteract chronic stress, which may be causing weight loss due to toxic reactions. (See Digestive Disorders.)

**Worms** can seriously compromise the body and interfere with proper digestion and assimilation, which leaves the body susceptible to poor skin and coat conditions. Unlike skin parasites, internal parasitic infestation can be deadly. Avoid chemical worming medications, which are so harsh they can permanently damage the sensitive linings of the digestive tract, especially of young animals.

Herbal worming can be successful if you follow the directions carefully. Often these products need to be administered along with fasting for optimum effect. Seek out products which contain herbs such as *Rhubarb Root* (especially effective against round and pinworms), *Cayenne* (helps eliminate eggs), *Barberry Root*, *Senna Leaves*, *Wormwood*, *Quassia Bark* (works well on giardia, found in water), *Black Walnut Hulls*, *Neem*, or *Bilva* herb. These are all excellent general preparations for eliminating worms. (See Digestive Disorders.)

# Grooming Techniques

Once you have addressed any underlying imbalances that resulted in your pet's skin and coat conditions, you can use topical treatments and grooming techniques to help reverse these symptoms more quickly. Regular grooming prevents infestation and encourages good skin and coat condition. Matted fur houses dirt and restricts air that is needed for tissue healing and encourages chronic skin irritation and infection. To decide which grooming techniques you should employ for your pet, you should first determine your pet's coat type.

**Smooth Coat** is fur that is short and fine. Some smooth-coated breeds include Boxer, Greyhound, and smooth-haired Dachshunds. Dogs with thicker, denser smooth coats include Rottweilers, Corgis, and Labs. Smooth-coated cat breeds include Domestic Shorthair and Siamese. This type of fur requires little maintenance. You do not need to use a comb or bristle brush on a daily basis. A hound glove or towel is often sufficient.

**Silky Coat** refers to dogs such as the Afghan, Cocker Spaniel, and Lhasa Apso. Persian and Himalayans are silky-coated cats. This type of fur mats easily and requires a few hours of maintenance per week. Frequent brushing with a slicker or wire bristle brush, followed by cutting out the matted areas and then combing the coat is the minimum care needed. Usually every few months, the undercoat also needs to be stripped.

**Wiry Coat** dogs are easy to spot. Their rough looking, but often silky fur is easy to care for. West Highland Terriers and Airedales are the most easily recognized wire-coated dogs. Recently, a mutant feline gene has produced the California Wire-Coated cat. These do not require frequent brushing or trimming, but need regular combing to avoid mats. The top-coat must be stripped and plucked every four months. Follow this grooming procedure with a bath. Alternatively, you can use clippers every two months to trim the coat and a pair of scissors to cut the fur around the eyes and ears.

**Non-Shedding Curly Coats** are found on Poodles, Kerry Blue or Beddington Terriers, Portuguese Water Spaniels, and Bichon Frisé. Dogs with this type of coat do not promote allergic reactions in people. Pets with non-shedding curly coats must be bathed and groomed regularly, and should be mechanically clipped and scissored every six weeks.

**Long Coats with Undercoat** occur in dog breeds such as German Shepherds, Collies, Sheepdogs, St. Bernards, and Newfoundlands, and in Himalayan cats. Pets with this type of coat require intensive grooming. Give these pets baths twice a year. After bathing remove the dense undercoat by parting the coat and using a wire bristle brush. Weekly brushings and untangling of the fur is also recommended. Some owners prefer to keep these coats short to reduce grooming difficulties. This is not recommended during months of weather extremes, especially if your pet is an outdoor pet, or spends at least one-half hour per day outside. The topcoat provides warmth in the winter and creates cooling during the warmer months. It will actually increase your pet's chances of heat stroke if you remove this protective outer layer, especially with dark-colored pets. The outer coat provides a layer of cooled air between the external environment and the pet's skin. Without this layer the undercoat and skin bakes, and the pet can quickly overheat.

## GROOMING EQUIPMENT

Professional grooming may be needed in certain situations, but all aspects of grooming can be done at home. There are several home kits containing mechanical clippers and video instructions, so it is not hard to groom your pet by yourself. You should have a wire bristle brush or slicker and a comb. A fine-tooth comb is beneficial for removing fleas or plant parts from the coat. Hound gloves (for smooth finishes) and carders (like a lamb wool brush) are specialized brushes. Your local pet shop probably has in stock all the tools you will need. Scissors with a rounded safety tip is used to trim around the eyes, ears, tail, or other sensitive parts. Keep tools in good repair and store them in a dry area to prevent rust. Tools that are not properly cared for make grooming more difficult. It can also hurt your pet when scissors are not sharp and pull the fur rather than cut it.

## USING A COMB

Combs should have rounded teeth, on the tip and shaft, to avoid tearing the fur or skin. Some combs have teeth that swivel around in their base and do a superior job with less pulling or tearing. To break up matted areas, insert a wide-toothed comb to the depth of the fur. Hold the fur down against the skin with your free hand to avoid pulling the skin painfully. Use a finer-toothed comb to separate the undercoat and remove any dead hair that is not firmly attached. When you encounter any resistance in the coat, remove the comb and work the knot or mat a little at a time with your fingers, scissors, or the comb until you have teased it apart. Follow this with the fine-tooth comb to remove fleas or plant parts embedded in the undercoat or close to the skin.

## USING A BRISTLE BRUSH

Bristle brushes will take care of most of your pet's grooming needs and are useful for finishing off and smoothing the coat after combing. Bristles should be long enough to reach through your pet's coat to the skin. For a smooth-coated pet, brush in the direction of the "lay" of the coat. Begin at the pet's head, working back towards the tail. Be sure to brush any feathering on the tail, belly, or legs. For long hair, brush gently against the lay of the coat. Push the brush into the coat and twist slightly against the natural growth, working in short strokes. Work one small section at a time. Never brush the entire coat against the lay or you will break hairs and possibly promote matting. Use your comb to clean out the bristles frequently during brushing.

## USING A CARDER

This type of wire-bristled brush consists of a rectangular board with short, bent wires mounted on it. This tool helps remove the loose, dead undercoat on shorter-haired pets. To use a carder on longer-haired breeds twist the carder towards the surface after working the teeth gently through to the skin.

## USING A HOUND GLOVE

Natural finishing bristles are mounted on a glove to groom shorthaired coats and give medium-coated breeds a finished look. This type of brush is very effective on shorthaired cats and is easier to use than brushes or combs. Grooming with a hound glove is so gentle the cat will think you are just petting them, not actually doing anything to them. Natural bristle gloves and gloves with rubber bumps on the surface can be used to massage tense pets and stimulate circulation, which supports detoxification and healing.

## BATHING YOUR PET

Do not bathe your pet too frequently. This can strip vital oils from the skin and create excessive production of oils to counter the dryness. Always remove tangles or mats prior to bathing, even if you plan to finish the grooming after the bath. You can give your pet a dry cornstarch shampoo whenever it is needed. The cornstarch will lift dirt to the surface and absorb odors. Simply sprinkle it on and work it into the coat, then brush out the coat well. Avoid chemicals, since the skin will absorb anything that is put on it.

Ask someone to help you bathe your pet. You can secure cats by putting them in a specially designed bag. Put cotton inside its ears first.

Use a high-quality organic cleaner formulated for your pet's needs. Wet the pet's back with warm water and work the water into the coat. Apply a little shampoo (less is best) and work it into a lather. Lather the whole body including the rear and the legs. Shampoo the head and face last, since most pets do not like this part. Rinse the pet thoroughly, starting at the head and working back. Shampoo that is left on your pet will irritate the skin and can cause rashes. Some finishing rinses, conditioners, or flea and tick dips should not rinsed off, but the shampoo should always be removed prior to these applications. Squeeze out excess water and towel dry. You can use a blow dryer, but introduce it to your pet slowly. Never apply it too close to the skin or leave it on too long.

## OTHER CROSSING PRESS PET BOOKS

**Bark Busters**

***Solving Your Dog's Behavioral Problems***

By Sylvia Wilson

This step-by-step guide will help you improve your relationship with your pet. The simple, effective techniques are designed to work together with a dog's natural instincts, without cruelty.

$12.95 • Paper • ISBN 0-89594-881-8

**The Holistic Puppy**

***How to Have a Happy, Healthy Dog***

By Diane Stein

Diane Stein shares her experience and gives useful information about choosing a dog and bringing it home, behavior training, handling and grooming, nutrition, and solving the dog's emotional problems.

$14.95 • Paper • ISBN 0-89594-946-6

**Natural Healing for Dogs and Cats**

By Diane Stein

This invaluable resource tells how to use nutrition, minerals, massage, herbs, homeopathy, acupuncture, acupressure, flower essences, and psychic healing for optimal health.

$16.95 • Paper • ISBN 0-89594-614-9

**The Natural Remedy Book for Dogs & Cats**

By Diane Stein

*An informative guide to the use of nutrition, vitamins, massage, herbs, and homeopathy to support your pet's health and vitality.*

—NAPRA Trade Journal

$16.95 • Paper • ISBN 0-89594-686-6

## OTHER CROSSING PRESS PET BOOKS

**Psycho Kitty?**
***Understanding Your Cat's Crazy Behavior***
By Pam Johnson-Bennett

Is your cat's behavior making you crazy? Johnson-Bennett believes that trying to understand how your cat thinks is a key to your cat's misbehavior. She shares real cases to illustrate various problems and explains how she arrives at an appropriate solution through behavior modification.

$12.95 • Paper • ISBN 0-89594-909-1

**Twisted Whiskers**
***Solving Your Cat's Behavior Problems***
By Pam Johnson

Johnson's cat-friendly, no-nonsense techniques glow with common sense and insight...a practical guide and an inspiration.

$12.95 • Paper • ISBN 0-89594-710-2

To receive a current catalog from The Crossing Press please call toll-free, 800-777-1048.

**www.crossingpress.com**